INTRODUCTION TO
THE HISTORY OF MEDICAL AND VETERINARY MYCOLOGY

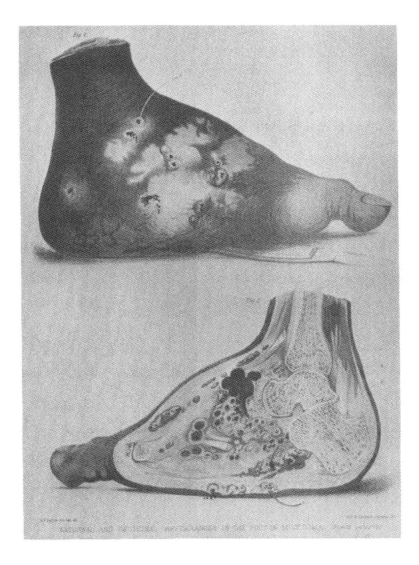

Black mycetoma of the foot (*Madurella mycetomatis*) (H. Vandyke Carter, 1874, pl. 2).

INTRODUCTION TO

THE HISTORY OF MEDICAL AND VETERINARY MYCOLOGY

G. C. AINSWORTH

Formerly Director of the Commonwealth Mycological Institute, Kew, UK

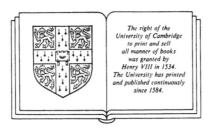

The right of the
University of Cambridge
to print and sell
all manner of books
was granted by
Henry VIII in 1534.
The University has printed
and published continuously
since 1584.

CAMBRIDGE UNIVERSITY PRESS

Cambridge

London   New York   New Rochelle

Melbourne   Sydney

PUBLISHED BY THE PRESS SYNDICATE OF THE UNIVERSITY OF CAMBRIDGE
The Pitt Building, Trumpington Street, Cambridge, United Kingdom

CAMBRIDGE UNIVERSITY PRESS
The Edinburgh Building, Cambridge CB2 2RU, UK
40 West 20th Street, New York NY 10011–4211, USA
477 Williamstown Road, Port Melbourne, VIC 3207, Australia
Ruiz de Alarcón 13, 28014 Madrid, Spain
Dock House, The Waterfront, Cape Town 8001, South Africa

http://www.cambridge.org

First published 19 March 1987
First paperback edition 2002

A catalogue record for this book is available from the British Library

Library of Congress Cataloguing in Publication data
Ainsworth, G. C. (Geoffrey Clough), 1905–
Introduction to the history of medical and veterinary mycology.
Bibliography.
Includes indexes.
1. Medical mycology – History.   2. Veterinary mycology – History.
I. Title. [DNLM: 1. Mycoses – history.
2. Mycoses – veterinary. QW 11.1 A279ia]
RC117.A54   1986   616.9'69   86-9619

ISBN 0 521 30715 5 hardback
ISBN 0 521 52455 5 paperback

To the memory of
CHESTER WILSON EMMONS
(1900–85)
Chief Medical Mycologist
National Institutes of Health
Bethesda, Maryland, USA
(1936–66)

CONTENTS

PREFACE

Although possessing deep, if slender, roots that can be traced back to ancient times, medical and veterinary mycology is essentially a development of the twentieth century, especially the past fifty years during which several mycoses at first considered to be rarities have been shown to affect millions of men, women, and children and their domesticated animals. Much has been established regarding the epidemiology of fungus infections of man and animals and the whole field has been increasingly well documented by textbooks, monographs, and reviews of 'recent advances' in many branches of the subject. These last, because of the short time scale, often provide historical summaries which give specialists access to detailed information not covered by this introductory survey. Here the attempt made to sketch in the historical background by illustrating the approaches to a series of basic problems is limited to what may be described as the 'natural history' of human and animal mycoses. The next step, the investigation of the host–pathogen interaction at the cellular and molecular level, already well advanced for some other infections of man, although begun for mycopathology is only hinted at. As parallel developments, attention is also given to fungus allergy and poisoning by fungi, especially mycotoxicoses resulting from the inadvertent consumption of moulded human food or animal feed.

January 1986   G.C.A.

ACKNOWLEDGEMENTS

Writing this history has increased my indebtedness to a number of friends, especially Peter K. C. Austwick, Roland W. Davies, the late Philip H. Gregory, Donald W. R. Mackenzie, and Phyllis M. Stockdale. Libero Ajello, Carroll W. Dodge, Dorothea Frey, Silver Keeping, Masahiko Okudaira, Juan E. Mackinnon, Mary P. Marples, and F. M. Rush-Munro all responded to requests for regional information and my wife read successive drafts and helped me with the indexing and proofs.

I am grateful for access to material in the sixteen public and institutional libraries visited and for the help so generously given me by the Wellcome Institute for the History of Medicine and the Commonwealth Mycological Institute.

For permission to use quotations I am indebted to the *Archives of Dermatology*, to re-work passages from my own writings to the British Mycological Society, the British Society for Mycopathology, and Pitman Publishing Ltd, and to reproduce illustrations to the following copyright holders or owners of the originals copied: Academic Press Inc., Fig. 32; *Archives of Dermatology*, Fig. 14; P. K. C. Austwick, Figs 3, 22, 30; *British Journal of Dermatology*, Figs 10, 28; Blackwell Scientific Publications Ltd, Fig. 41; Charlotte C. Campbell, Figs 50, 52; Commonwealth Mycological Institute, Figs 7, 18; R. W. Davies, Figs 39, 40; E. Drouhet, Figs 9, 53, 54; ISHAM, Fig. 16; Leicester University Press, Fig. 24; Linnean Society, Fig. 21; London School of Hygiene & Tropical Medicine, Fig. 5; Mycological Reference Laboratory, PHLS, Figs 11, 12, 34, 37, 46; *Mycopathologia*, Fig. 49; New York Academy of Science, Fig. 26; Nottingham University, Fig. 31; Photography Unit, NY State Dept of Health, Fig. 36; R. Vanbreuseghem, Fig. 47; Wellcome Institute for the History of Medicine Library, Figs 8, 27; Wellcome Museum of Medical Science, Fig. 51A.

1

Introduction

Medical and veterinary mycology (or 'mycopathology' as it is sometimes not very happily designated) is, essentially, the study of infectious disease in man and higher animals caused by fungi but, traditionally, it also includes diseases caused by actinomycetes (because these filamentous bacteria were at one time frequently classified as fungi) and allergic conditions induced by fungi and actinomycetes. During the past twenty-five years the foundations of medical and veterinary mycology have been completed and although in future knowledge of recognized mycoses will deepen, the relative importance of different mycoses will vary, and additional mycoses will be described, such developments should do little to disturb the relationship of this field to human and veterinary medicine in general. This would, therefore, appear to be an appropriate moment at which to pause and survey the history of a speciality which involved the collaboration of clinicians and pathologists with non-medically trained mycologists, microbiologists, and biochemists[1] (see Notes on the Text, pp. 171–80) before satisfactory progress could be made in the solution of many medical and veterinary problems.

That some larger fungi are poisonous (or hallucinogenic) for man has been on record for two thousand years but during the last few decades the recognition that many microfungi produce toxins (*mycotoxins*) in animal feed and human food which induce widespread and sometimes fatal disease in farm animals and man has resulted in the emergence of a major new branch of mycology (see Chapter 8. Cross-references without pagination may be elucidated via the Subject Index). Fungal infections of man, which are usually less-spectacular than poisonings, have been less frequently documented.

Possibly the earliest record of a mycotic infection is that in the Indian Atharva Veda [*c.* 2000–1000 BC] of mycetoma of the foot which was differentiated from filarial elephantitis of the foot and described under the name 'padavalmika' (foot-ant-hill), a forerunner of '*Fourmilière des vers*' (ant-hill of worms) used for the same condition by a French missionary at Ponticherry in 1714.[2]

Two mycoses familiar today – thrush[3] in infants and favus – were noted in the Greek and Roman classics. In the Hippocratic writings [5th century BC] thrush was included among references to aphthae and Aulus Cornelius Celsus [1st century AD] in *De re medicina* (Book vi (2)), following the nomenclature of Hippocrates, dealt with thrush under ulcers where he wrote:

...the most dangerous of these ulcers which the Greeks call aphthae, certainly in children; in them they often cause death, but there is not the same danger for men and women. These ulcers begin from the gums; next they invade the palate and the whole of the mouth, then they pass downwards to the ulva and throat, and if these are involved it is not easy for the child to recover. But the disease is even worse in a suckling, there is less possibility of its conquest by any remedy...[4]

In Book v of the same work Celsus drew attention to the boggy inflammatory lesions of some ringworm infections – the condition known ever since as 'the kerion of Celsus' – and in Book vi described favus:

...the condition is called porrigo, when between the hairs something like small scales rise up and become detached from the scalp: and at times they are moist, much more often dry. Sometimes this happens without ulceration, sometimes there is localized ulceration, and from this comes sometimes a foul odour, sometimes none. This generally occurs on the scalp, more seldom the beard, occasionally even on the eyebrow.[5]

In the centuries which followed the term 'porrigo' was used to cover various skin disorders and the Latin 'tinea'[6] was applied in a generic sense to ringworm (from a fanciful resemblance of the signs of the disease to the depredations of the clothes moth (*Tineola biselliella*)) which was recorded with increasing frequency.

There are records of the Tudors granting licences under the signet for loyal sufferers from ringworm to remain covered in the king's presence and on other ceremonial occasions and Samuel Pepys in his diary for 17 June 1665 recorded thrush as one of the terminal symptoms of Admiral Sir John Lawson. During the last decade of the seventeenth century the English antiquary John Aubry compared fairy rings and ringworm:

As to the green circles on the downes, vulgarly called faiery circles (dances), I presume they are generated from the breathing out of a fertile subterranean vapour. (The ring-worme on a man's flesh is circular. Excogitate a paralolisme between the cordial heat and ye subterranean heat, to elucidate the phaenomenon.)[7]

A pertinent comparison in spite of his incorrect explanation tinged with the doctrine of humours.

About the same time Sir William Dampier, when voyaging round the world, wrote in his journal after a visit to the Phillipines in 1686:

The *Mindanao* People are much troubled with a sort of Leprosie, the same as we observed in *Guam*. This Distemper runs with a dry scurf all over their Bodies, and causeth great itching in those that have it, making them frequently scratch and scrub themselves, which raiseth the outer Skin in small whitish flakes, like the scales of little Fish, when they are raised on end by a Knife. This makes their skin extraordinary rough...[8]

The same disease was subsequently observed in Polynesia and became known as 'Tokelau Itch' or 'Tokelau Disease', after the islands where the disorder was prevalent, but it was not until 1879 that one of the pioneers of tropical medicine, Patrick Manson, then Medical Officer to the Imperial Maritime Customs at Amoy, China, elucidated its aetiology. Manson noted the presence of mycelium in the skin scales and by experimental inoculation of one of his Chinese assistants showed the fungus to be the cause of the disease which he called 'tinea imbricata', because the skin scales appeared to be like overlapping tiles. Finally, in 1896, the French worker Raphael Blanchard named the fungus *Trichophyton concentricum* after the concentric patterns it caused on infected skin.

Tinea has been illustrated by a number of the old masters. In Murrillo's [1617–82] painting in the Hermandad de la Santa Carida, Seville, of St Elizabeth of Hungary washing the head of a child with another standing by her side scratching himself both children appear to be suffering from favus (Fig. 1)[9] as does the boy being considered for admission to the Amsterdam Leprosy House in the painting by Ferdinand Bol [1616–90] in the Rijksmuseum. Since Biblical times favus and leprosy have been confused and some of the clinical dermatology in *Leviticus* 13 could possibly be interpreted as an attempt at the differential diagnosis of these two conditions.[10]

During the eighteenth century and early years of the nineteenth a number of mycoses of higher animals were reported. On 12 May 1748, Henry Baker communicated to the Royal Society of London a letter he had recently received from the Norwich naturalist William Arderon describing observations on a fatal distemper that was certainly 'salmon disease' (saprolegniosis) affecting a roach (*Leuciscus rutilus*) in captivity. '...after this Fish has been a little while confined, the finny Part of its Tail begins to drop off Piece by Piece; and when the finny Part is all gone, a sort of

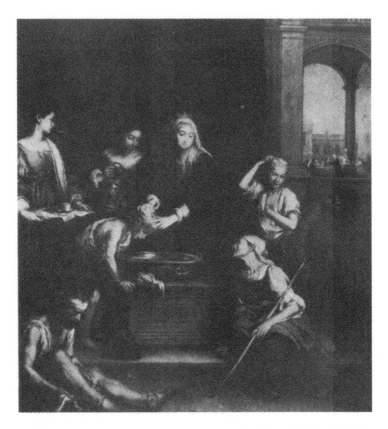

Fig. 1. 'St Elizabeth of Hungary caring for the sick' by Murillo. (Hospital Santa Caridad, Seville).

Mortification seizes upon the Tail itself, and gradually creeps along until it reaches the Intestines, at which time the Fish immediately dies'; so wrote Arderon who also described the 'fine fibrillous Substance' which grew out from the mortified tissues (Fig. 2). The same condition, but in a goldfish (*Cyprinus auratus*) was reported by J. Hughes Bennett to the Royal Society of Edinburgh in 1842 (Bennett, 1844). Records of avian aspergillosis began in 1749 with the observation on the moulding of incubating eggs by the versatile René de Réaumur (inventor of the eighty-degree thermometer scale) in *The art of hatching and bringing up of domestic fowls of all kinds...*, the description of a 'mould or blue mucor' in the thoracic air sac of a Scaup duck (*Aythya marila*) by Montagu (1813), and a similar condition in a jay (*Garrulus glandarius*) by Mayer (1815) followed. Subsequently, the English anatomist Richard Owen when dissecting a

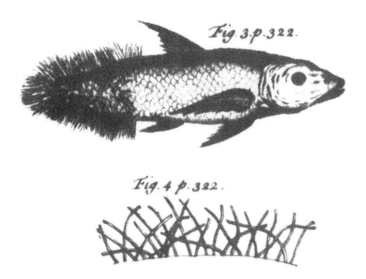

Fig. 2. Saprolegniosis in a roach. (W. Arderon, 1748).

flamingo (*Phaenicopteris ruber*) found 'a green vegetable mould or *mucor*' in the lungs, recognized the parasitic relationship, and concluded 'that internal parasites are not derived exclusively from the animal kingdom' and 'that there are *Entophyta* as well as *Entozoa*' (Owen, 1832). Concurrently, James Kerr, a retired veterinary surgeon of the First Bengal Light Cavalry, described in the *Veterinarian* for 1829 a disease of horses of unknown cause characterized by ulceration of the angle of the lip, face, scrotum, and legs under the name of 'bausette' (or 'bursattee' of which there are a dozen variant spellings). During the next 45 years there were additional communications on the disease to the same journal from veterinary officers of cavalry and artillery regiments stationed in India and others speculating on the cause of the condition, the occurrence of which was associated with water and wet weather. One notable contribution was that in 1874 by F. F. Collins who concluded 'that an active foreign agent is in existence to produce appearance so peculiar, and I do not know of an agent capable of producing such peculiarities other than that of a parasitic origin, and that parasite I conceive to be of vegetable organization...'[11]. From 1886 bursattee was recognized in the United States as 'leeches', 'Florida horse leech' (because of the belief that leeches were responsible), and 'swamp cancer' and in 1895 P.A. Fish of the Division of Animal Pathology of the US Bureau of Animal Industry in addition to an interesting historical review of the condition illustrated

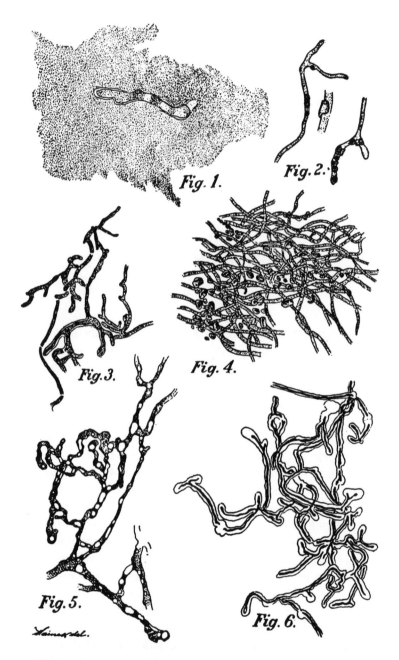

Fig. 3. Fungus from the lip of a horse affected by hyphomycosis. (Fish, 1895).

elements of an unidentified fungus in preparations from infected lips (Fig. 3). The next major studies were made by Haan & Hoogamer (1903) in the Dutch East Indies who named the disease 'Hyphomycosis destruens equi' and Witkamp (1924) called the pathogen by the illegitimate name 'Hyphomyces equi'. Subsequently Bridges & Emmons (1961) suggested that the pathogen was a phycomycete which Austwick & Copland (1974), on the basis of cultures from four cases of 'swamp cancer' in Papua New Guinea concluded was a species of *Pythium*.

The concept of pathogenicity

No real progress in the understanding of mycotic disease could be made until the concept of pathogenicity had been established and that took some two hundred years. Robert Hooke, the young versatile Curator of Experiments of the Royal Society of London, in his *Micrographia*, 1665, illustrated rose rust (*Phragmidium mucronatum*), the Frenchman Isaac Bénedict Prévost (in 1807) offered experimental proof that bunt of wheat was caused by *Tilletia tritici*, and in 1835 an Italian lawyer turned farmer, Agostino Bassi, demonstrated that the muscardine disease of silkworms was caused by a fungus (subsequently named in his honour *Beauveria bassiana*). In spite of these findings, the pathogenicity of fungi to plants and animals was not generally accepted until after the mid-nineteenth century. This was in large measure due to the question of pathogenicity becoming associated with spontaneous generation and heterogenesis (the origination of new organisms from living cells of a different species) which also proved to be intractable problems. The story of their elucidation has often been told – never better than by Bulloch (1938) in his history of bacteriology – so that only the briefest summary is necessary here. As late as 1642, Jean Baptiste von Helmont [1577–1644] believed that adult mice originated spontaneously from bran and old rags. Francisco Redi [1626–98] in 1668 demonstrated that maggots in rotten meat originated from eggs laid by flies and not *de novo* as hitherto supposed. Subsequently, the fundamental researches of the Abbot Lazzaro Spallanzani [1729–99] in Italy during the seventeen-sixties, Franz Schulz [1815–74] and Theodore Schwann [1810–82] in Germany, and finally those of Pasteur [1822–95] in France in the early eighteen-sixties and concurrently John Tyndall [1820–93] and William Roberts [1830–99] in England provided irrefutable evidence that neither spontaneous generation nor heterogenesis of micro-organisms occurs although some proponents of the latter, such as H. C. Bastian

[1837–1915], remained unconvinced and carried the heresy over into the twentieth century (in *The origin of life*, 1913).

The beginning of medical mycology as a distinct branch of medicine can be precisely dated as 1842 to 1844, the years during which David Gruby in Paris published a series of six short, but outstanding, papers in which he showed, very convincingly, that four types of ringworm and also thrush were mycotic in origin (see Chapter 2).

The reception of Gruby's findings varied from enthusiastic acceptance to disbelief (see Chapter 4). Bacterial infections being as yet unrecognized, a fungal origin for cholera and other bacterial diseases was widely claimed but after Koch's classical work on anthrax in 1876 and his demonstrations of the true nature of tuberculosis and cholera during 1882–83, the major importance of bacteria as agents of disease in man and animals became established and pathogenic fungi suffered eclipse. Study of ringworm did continue and this was given a major impetus by the researches of the French dermatologist Raimond Sabouraud which began in the early eighteen-nineties and culminated in the publication of his important monograph, *Les Teignes*, 1910. Another complicating factor before the introduction of pure culture techniques by Koch and others[12] was the phenomenon of pleomorphism (in its original connotation of the existence of sexual and asexual states of one fungus) and the life cycles of fungi in which some workers included both diverse mycelial species and yeasts – and even bacteria. This led to the fantasies of Ernst Hallier (see Chapter 4), assistant professor of botany at Jena, whose claims were finally authoritatively discredited by his fellow countryman the eminent mycologist Anton de Bary. In the late eighteen-seventies medical mycology received a major addition resulting from investigations by German workers on actinomycosis in cattle and in man; the bacteriologist Bollinger coining the designation 'lumpy jaw' (1871) for the cattle disease while his botanical colleague Harz introduced the binomial *Actinomyces bovis* (1877) for the pathogen. Bollinger and Harz had before them both actinomycosis (lumpy jaw) and actinobacillosis (wooden tongue) of cattle caused by the bacterium *Actinobacillus lignieresii*. These two conditions, which have been much confused, were first clearly distinguished by Lignières & Spitz (1902) but the genus *Actinobacillus* was not proposed until 1910, by Brumpt.

At the turn of the century, protozoologists made what eventually proved to be even more important additions to mycopathology. In 1892, Alejandro Posadas, an undergraduate student of Robert Wernicke in Buenos Aires, first described the 'protozoon' believed to be responsible for 'mycosis fungoides' (Fig. 4) and four years later the same organism was inde-

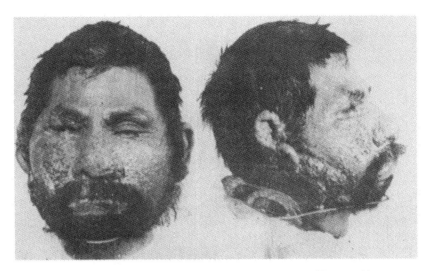

Fig. 4. Specimen at the Faculty of Medicine, University of Buenos Aires from Posadas and Wernicke's original case of coccidioidomycosis. (Niño, 1950).

pendently described in California where it was named *Coccidioides immitis* by Rixford & Gilchrist (1896) after consultation with the eminent proto-zoologist C. W. Stiles. Eight years later Ophuls & Moffitt (1900) recognized that the protozoan was the pathogenic phase of a mycelial fungus. In 1906, the American S. T. Darling when stationed at the Ancon Hospital, Panama Canal Zone, described *Histoplasma capsulatum* (Fig. 5) but in this case it was twenty-eight years before the fungal nature of the pathogen was demonstrated independently and almost simultaneously by De-Monbreun (1934) and Hansmann & Schencken (1934) in the United States. Subsequent studies on these two widespread systemic mycoses probably did more to establish the relevance and importance of medical and veterinary mycology than any other investigations (see Chapter 5).

It is an acceptable generalization that up to the First World War the fungi causing mycoses in man and animals were studied by medical men and veterinarians who were self-taught mycologists and not by specialists in the study of fungi whose rare excursions into the medical field were notably unsuccessful. As a result, much that was published on these pathogenic fungi was not in line with mycological practice and this led mycologists to regard these pathogens as a special group, 'medical fungi', of dubious relationships. Although a few non-medically trained mycolo-gists in France and elsewhere took up the study of medical fungi,

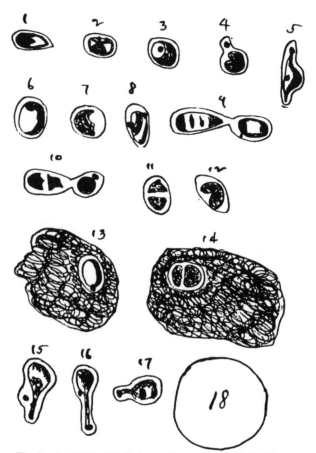

Fig. 1.—(× 2000), 1 to 8, forms of parasite; 9, 10, 11, 12 manner of subdivision; 13, 14, parasites within nuclei of spleen cells; 15, 16, 17, flagellate forms; 18, alveolar epithelial cell containing parasites.

Fig. 5. First illustration of *Histoplasma capsulatum*. (Darling, 1906).

developments in North America during the nineteen-thirties transformed the mycopathological scene. It was in the United States that a series of highly trained young mycologists were appointed to posts in the Department of Health, universities, and hospitals where they could work in close collaboration with clinicians and it soon became apparent that the major differential character of 'medical fungi' was pathogenicity to man and higher animals. They exhibited sexual and asexual phases and could be satisfactorily characterized without reference to their pathogenicity. Much confused taxonomy was elucidated and the corresponding nomenclature given greater precision. In addition, a number of up to then rare pathogenic fungi (and also others including some ringworm fungi) were isolated with increasing frequency from soil, animal dung, and other substrata and the conclusion reached that many of the fungi causing mycoses are what has come to be termed 'opportunistic'; that is, they establish themselves as pathogens only when a subject is by chance exposed to an exceptionally high concentration of their spores or when the subjects are 'compromised', that is their immunity is decreased by another disease, for example diabetes, or by treatment with antibiotics, immunosuppressants, etc., such as that which precedes organ transplantation. In marked contrast to plant pathogens, few if any fungi pathogenic to man and higher animals are dependent on a host for survival. They are able to grow saprobicly and regarding their nutritional requirements it is interesting to note that, in marked contrast to bacteria, these have been shown to be less exacting for the highly pathogenic than for the weakly pathogenic.[13] Another major distinction between mycotic disease in plants and animals is due to the possession of an immune system by the latter so that serological techniques may be employed to detect current and past infections, in therapy and preventative treatment, and also for the identification of the pathogens.

Treatment of mycotic disease like that of disease in general has shown extreme diversity over the centuries and much, especially early, therapy was irrational if tempered by the empirical approach of practising physicians, which tends to promote the survival of regimes which appear to be the more successful or meet the patients' expectations. Only recently have therapeutic agents, including antibiotics, been derived from laboratory investigations.

After an overenthusiastic acceptance of fungi as the cause of infectious disease in man and animals followed by a period of neglect and then one of what might be called confusion, the last fifty years have seen the relationship of mycopathology to medicine and veterinary science firmly established. It is now clear that while fungi are the principal cause of disease in plants they play a relatively minor, if still significant, role in diseases of man and higher animals. Forty years ago Chester Emmons wrote:

In *Vital Statistics of the United States for 1942*, 1,385,187 deaths were reported. Of these 359 were attributed to fungi. This is less than 0.03% of the total, but in this registration area it is nearly twice as many as the total of known deaths due to paratyphoid fever, undulant fever, smallpox, rabies, leprosy, plague, cholera, yellow fever, and relapsing fever together; it is greater than the number due to all the typhus-like diseases together; and it is more than half the number due to either typhoid, tetanus, or poliomyelitis. In fairness in comparison it should be pointed out that many of these better known diseases rarely cause death, because of effective prophylactic and control measures.[14]

and the position is much the same today.

Some mycotic diseases of the skin and superficial tissues of worldwide incidence are at least a costly inconvenience – the annual expenditure on medicaments for ringworm infections in the United States during the nineteen-sixties and seventies has been estimated as 25 million dollars[15] – and a number of widespread, if more localized, systematic mycoses have an incidence measured in millions where they are endemic. Both superficial and systematic mycoses may prove chronic or fatal because of therapeutic deficiencies, but fungi are unlikely to compete in importance with bacteria and viruses as disease-inducing agents in man and his domesticated animals. Many fungi are typically only potentially pathogenic, they are saprobes of man's environment able under favourable circumstances to cause disease and this possibility is one that should always be borne in mind when investigating a condition of unknown aetiology.

2

Aetiology: dermatophytes and the taxonomic problem

Although clinicians, both medical and veterinary, have of necessity to prescribe treatment (which may be successful) for conditions of unknown aetiology the first step in the rational approach to an infectious disease is the determination of the causal agent and its correct taxonomic assignment which allows the findings of different workers to be compared and integrated. Among those who first demonstrated the fungal origin of mycotic disease in man one name is outstanding, that of David Gruby, who showed thrush and different manifestations of ringworm to be caused by different fungi and a chronological summary of the taxonomic approach to dermatophytes – which with the pathogenic yeasts (see Chapter 4) still constitute the two main areas of mycopathological endeavour – well illustrates most of the mycological problems that had to be resolved before a relatively stable classification could be achieved.

David Gruby[1]

David Gruby (Fig. 6), son of a poor Jewish farmer, was born at Kis-Kèr in South Hungary [now Bačko Dobro Polje, Yugoslavia] on 20 August 1810. He left home at the age of fifteen, acquired an education which enabled him to work his way through the university, first at Pest, then Vienna where he studied medicine and gained a doctorate in 1839 for his thesis *Observationes microscopicae ad morphologiam* which was published the next year as a book intended to be the first part of a handbook on microscopical pathology. He was offered a professorship by the University of Vienna on the condition that he became a Catholic. This was unacceptable so after deliberation he decided to settle in Paris (then the leading centre of medical research) where later he was again unsuccessful in obtaining a post either at the University or the Veterinary College at Alfort. He made the move in 1840 and in 1841 started a private research laboratory where he also offered instruction on the microscopy of normal and pathological specimens to, among others, François Magendie, Claude Bernard,

13

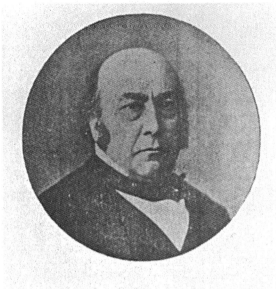

LE DOCTEUR GRUBY A SOIXANTE ANS

Fig. 6. David Gruby (1810–98).

O. Delaford (professor at the Veterinary School, Alfort), and Frederic Berg. Concurrently he worked at the Foundling Hospital, under the pediatrician Jacques François Baron, where he must have become familiar with both thrush and ringworm. He also knew of Bassi's elucidation of the mycotic nature of muscardine disease of silkworms and this too must have been one of the stimuli for the series of six short unillustrated papers on ringworm and thrush published in the *Comptes Rendus* of the Académie des Sciences between 1841 and 1844 by which Gruby will always be remembered by mycopathologists.

Gruby published nothing more on these mycoses but in 1844 he did publish a note on a mass of fungal growth found in the human stomach (Gruby, 1844b) and after his death among his papers were drawings dated 1848 showing that concretions from lacrimal ducts were composed of mycelium, later shown by others to be that of aerobic actinomycetes.[2] His research interests were wide ranging. One major discovery was the protozoan in the blood of frogs for which he proposed the genus *Trypanasoma* in 1844. He also observed, for the first time, microfilaria in dogs and transmitted the infection from one dog to another by blood transfusion. He studied dietetics, anaesthesia (urging that experiments on living animals should only be carried out under an anaesthetic), contributed to the development of photomicroscopy, advocated the substitution of cotton for lint (brushed linen (flax)) in surgical and general medical use and, during the Franco-Prussian war, designed a collapsible hospital tent, a wheeled stretcher, and other first aid equipment. In 1854 he obtained a licence to practise medicine in France and for the rest of his life worked as a successful and much sought, if unorthodox, physician whose patients included such celebrities as Dumas *père* and *fils*, George Sand, Alphonse Daudet, Heine, and Chopin. With increasing age he became increasingly eccentric but was continually developing new interests such as medical meteorology and astronomy. One feature of Gruby the physician is difficult to understand. He 'stubbornly refused to recognize the importance of germs in different diseases, and in his later years he no longer believed in the value of vaccination'.[3] Gruby died, unmarried, in November 1898 in his eighty-ninth year.

Gruby on ringworm

Gruby's first communication (Gruby, 1841a) to the Paris Academy of Sciences, read on 12 July 1841, was on favus, 'la vrai teigne' as he called it. After reviewing briefly the opinions of representative dermatologists on the nature of the condition and its site and on the unsatisfactory nature of the characteristics for its diagnosis based on the site and appearance of the scutula ('croûtes'), whether contagious, and the odour, he offered more precise criteria. He began:

To recognize the true teigne one has to examine under the microscope, at a magnification of 300, a small piece of the crust crushed in a drop of water between two glass slides. One will then see a large quantity of round or oblong corpuscles [microconidia]... In addition to this are observed small septate filaments [hyphae]...

for which he gives the measurements.[4] A description of the scutulum and its relation to the skin and hair then follows.

The climate of opinion was favourable for the elucidation of the aetiology of ringworm and, unknown to Gruby, Professor Johannes Lukes Schönlein of Berlin, stimulated by Bassi's work on the muscardine disease of silkworms, had already, in 1839, noted the 'vegetable' nature of favus. In a second communication (in the form of a letter, Gruby 1841b) to the Academy, made three weeks after the first, Gruby critically discusses Schönlein's findings and supplements his own account of favus by reporting the results of inoculation experiments. In his first experiment on humans Gruby inoculated the arm of Professor Rinneker of Wurzburg when a slow inflammation with slight suppuration followed and he subsequently inoculated himself four times with similar results. Inoculation of 24 silkworms, six reptiles, four birds, and eight mammals were negative. Inoculation of 30 phanerogamic plants resulted in one infection but no details, nor the identity of the plant, are given.

Gruby did not name the favus pathogen and this requirement was met by a third independent discoverer of the nature of favus, Robert Remak,[5] a Polish Jew, born in Poznan (then part of Prussia) in 1815, for whom, as for Gruby, his faith and nationality proved life-long hindrances. At the age of eighteen he moved to Berlin (where he lived for the rest of his life) and there, while working under S. F. Barez [1790–1856] at the Charité Hospital he discovered that favus scutula were composed of spherical bodies and ramified fibres. He allowed this observation to be published in 1837 in the doctoral thesis, De morbo scropuloso, of Xaver Hube, a fellow Polish student. Remak did not realize that he had seen a fungus. Schönlein's publication gave him the clue and in 1842 he published an account of the successful inoculation of his own left forearm. He also grew the fungus on slices of apple. In 1843 he became an assistant in Schönlein's Clinic and two years later in his important Diagnostische und pathogenetische Untersuchungen . . . of 1845 reporting his investigations at the Clinic he named the favus fungus, in a new genus, as Achorion schoenleinii in honour of Professor Schönlein but this name is antedated by the Oidium schoenleinii of H. Lebert, published in France earlier in the same year, of which Remak's name is usually taken to be a transfer.

Gruby's next communication to the Academy (Gruby, 1842a) was a demonstration of the fungal nature of thrush in children (a discovery made independently by Langenbeck (1839) and Frederic T. Berg (1841); the latter by then Professor of Pediatrics in Stockholm had attended Gruby's classes in Paris. This was followed later in the year (Gruby, 1842b) by the results of his study of 'phytomentagra' (ringworm of the beard, tinea barbae) which he showed to be caused by an ectothrix trichophyton. He clearly described how microscopical examination of a hair:

reveals that its entire dermal portion is enveloped by cryptogams forming a vegetable layer between the hair sheath and the hair proper, so that the hair is enclosed in a sheath formed exclusively by the cryptogams, like the finger of a glove.

and he compared the 'mentagrophytes' with the cryptogams causing favus and thrush.[6] Again Gruby did not name these two pathogens. That was left to the versatile microscopist Charles Robin (Fig. 7) who in his

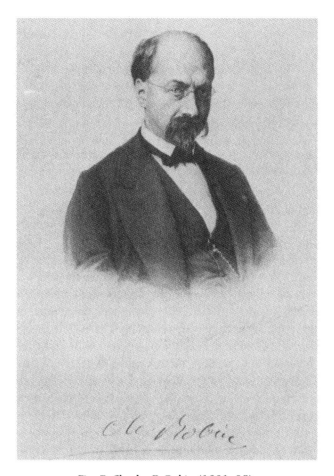

Fig. 7. Charles P. Robin (1821–85).

Histoire naturelle des végétaux parasites qui croissent sur l'homme et des animaux, 1853 (an expansion of his doctoral thesis of 1847), proposed the names *Oidium albicans* and *Microsporon mentagrophytes*.

Gruby then turned his attention to 'porrigo decalvans' or 'phyto-alopécie', as he called it (Gruby, 1843), in which the infected hair is coated by a small-spored cryptogam which he named, after Victor Audouin of the Paris Natural History Museum for his work on muscardine disease, '*Microsporum audouini*'. The only subsequent modification of this name has been the trivial correction to the latinization of the specific epithet so that *Microsporum audouinii* is the oldest name still current for a fungus pathogenic for man. It was in this paper that Gruby distinguished

'maladies parasitiques végétales, or 'phytoparasites' as a new class of
diseases for 'teigne faveuse', 'phytomentagre', 'phytoalopécie' and
'muguet'.[7]

Finally the series was completed by a report (Gruby, 1844a) on tinea
tonsurans of Mahon, herpes tonsurans of Cazenave or (in Gruby's nomenclature) 'rizo-phyto-alopécia' in which the pathogen causes an endothrix
type of infection.[8]

By careful microscopic examination of hair fragments of tinea tonsurans, one
recognizes that their entire tissue is filled by cryptogams and that the hairs are still
covered by their epidermal scales, when their interior is already filled with spores.

This fungus was the *Trichophyton tonsurans* described by P. H. Malmsten
of Stockholm in 1845.

After Gruby

Gruby maintained a lifelong interest in microscopy in which he was expert.
(After his death more than 15 000 microscopic preparations and 2 000
photomicrographs were found among his possessions). His microscopical
descriptions of the four ringworm fungi were as good, or better, than those
of most authors for the next fifty years, although he did interpret both ecto-
and endothrix trichophyton infections as developing upwards from the
hair bulb whereas the invading fungus grows downwards towards the
bulb as the hair elongates. His clinical descriptions were less satisfactory.
It was unfortunate that he associated both microsporosis and endothrix
trichophyton infections with alopecia, a non-parasitic baldness, and he did
not even indicate that children are those most frequently infected by *M.
audouinii*. This introduced a confusion which induced some to discredit
Gruby's work (see Chapter 4) which was, however, welcomed by others;
as, for example, by J. H. Bennett of Edinburgh who in 1842 confirmed
Gruby's elucidation of favus (and observed favus [*Trichophyton quinckeanum*] in mice) although he concluded after unsuccessful attempts to
inoculate himself, that the vegetations associated with pathological states
'always arise in living animals *previously* diseased' (Bennett, 1844). This
conclusion was subsequently abandoned after one of the gentleman in
attendance at Bennett's polyclinical class at the Royal Dispensary Edinburgh during the summer of 1845 volunteered to permit his arm to be
inoculated when typical favus spots developed (Bennett, 1858:799).

One problem for many of those who accepted the pathogenicity of the
fungi associated with ringworm was: Were there many fungi or was there
only one? For example, J. Lowe of Edinburgh concluded that *Trichophyton
tonsurans* was a spore form of the favus fungus and that both were forms

of *Aspergillus glaucus* (Lowe, 1858); a conclusion with which the Rev. M. J. Berkeley, the leading British mycologist at the time, concurred.[9] This difficulty was in part due to the different dermatophytes in skin or, to a less extent, hair appearing similar to the casual observer, in part to the primitive state of culture techniques and the failure to ensure the purity of the cultures, and in part to the mycological discoveries concurrently being made in France by the Tulasne brothers who in the three volumes of their important *Selecta fungorum carpologia*, 1861–5, were able to show in convincing detail that apparently unrelated ascospore-producing and conidia-producing fungi were in reality the sexual and asexual states of one fungus; states which became known as the 'perfect' and 'imperfect' or, in current terminology, the *teleomorphic* and *anamorphic*. Less meticulous workers, and particularly Professor Ernst Hallier (who in 1865 claimed that the favus fungus was a phase of *Penicillium glaucum*) frequently involved bacteria and fungi in one supposed life cycle. Yeasts, being such common contaminants, were also invoked. In 1863, *Skin diseases of parasitic origin...including the description and relations of the fungi found in man* by Tilbury Fox, a 27-year-old London dermatologist, was published. This book, the first in England on fungi of medical importance, contains little original mycology; Fox acknowledges his indebtedness to Küchenmeister's *Die in und an dem Körper des lebenden Menschen vorkommenden Parasiten*, 1855 (an English translation of which had appeared in 1857), for descriptions of the various fungi and its chief interest lies in the presentation of the evidence that there was but one essential fungus (Fig. 8) – in Fox's opinion *Torula* sensu Turpin (yeasts such as *Torulopsis* and *Saccharomyces*), at least as far as the mucedinous fungi were concerned for he was 'most desirous not to ride any hobby'. Not everyone, however, was convinced. As Thomas Hillier pointed out, '...these facts do not...prove the identity of fungi...they seem to show that a soil which is favourable for one fungus may encourage the growth of another distinct fungus' and Thomas McCall Anderson in 1861 had recognized four cutaneous affections of the skin (favus, tinea tonsurans, pityriasis versicolor, and, following Gruby, as he thought, alopecia areata) each of which he believed to be due to the presence of a distinct fungus. In the United Kingdom it was George Thin who showed by careful cultural work on a variety of liquid media and on the 'meat-gelatine' recently introduced by Koch that *Trichophyton tonsurans* is a fungus in its own right 'totally distinct from the common fungi whose spores infest all the objects by which we are surrounded' (Thin, 1881, 1887). Similar cultural work was done at the Pasteur Institute in Paris by Duclaux (1886) and Verujski (1887) and this

176   ENTOPHYTES AND THEIR RELATIONS.

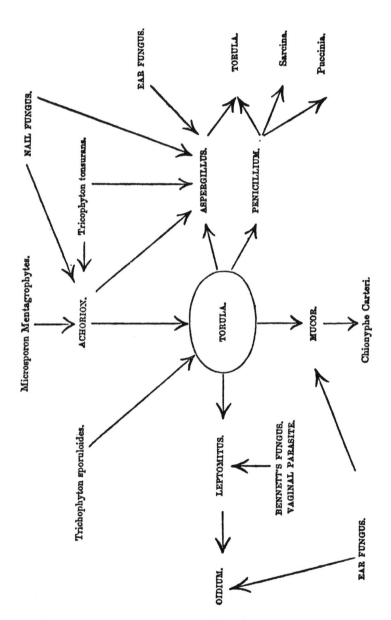

Fig. 8. Entophytes and their relations. (Tilbury Fox (1863): 176).

prepared the way for the suggestion by Furthmann & Neebe in 1891 that there was more than one *Trichophyton* fungus and for the now classical investigations by Sabouraud in France which established the plurality of the ringworm fungi beyond all doubt.

Sabouraud and ringworm

Raimond Jacques Andrieu Sabouraud[10] (Fig. 9) was born 24 November 1864 at Nantes into a family with a medical tradition. After education at Nantes he moved to Paris where, qualifying in medicine in 1890, he lived and worked until his death on 4 February 1938. He was a man of diverse talents – a practising sculptor, the author of a well received book on Montaigne – and became, and will remain, world-famous for his studies on ringworm and the dermatophytes begun at the suggestion of Ernst Besnier, the leading French dermatologist of the time. Sabouraud was well qualified for the project having studied bacteriology at the Pasteur Institute under Roux and so was able to make use of pure culture techniques in which for 37 years he was assisted by Paul Théveniau, who as a boy came to him as a patient suffering from a severe palada and entered his service to become both collaborator and friend until they both retired in 1929. Sabouraud's other strength was his skill as a clinician.

Sabouraud began his researches in 1892. He at once was able to distinguish two types of head ringworm in children by clinical appearance, microscopical examination, and culture as the tinea capitis with small spores and the tinea capitis with large spores and at the end of the year the first instalment of his 'Contribution à l'étude de la trichophytie humaine' appeared in the Parisian *Annales de dermatologie et de syphilographie* where he named the fungus associated with the first *Trichophyton microsporum*. Two years later, when preparing his doctoral thesis, *Les trichophyties humaines*, he read Gruby's papers and found that the same observations had been made fifty years before and that his *T. microsporum* was Gruby's *Microsporum audouinii*. More than sixty other publications followed in rapid succession and these were finally integrated in his 855-page monograph, *Les Teignes*, of 1910.

Sabouraud's method was to make a careful clinical examination, then to subject the infected hair or skin scale to microscopy, make a pure culture and to observe the cultural features under standard conditions on a range of standardized culture media, especially those based on what he called his 'test medium'. He compared 500 cultures on three variants of this

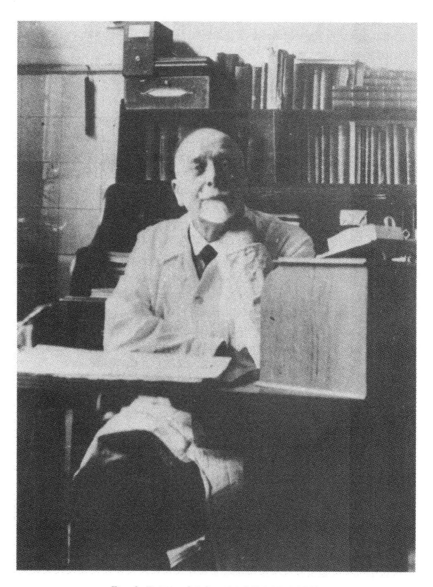

Fig. 9. Raimond Sabouraud (1864–1938).

medium containing different sugars and recognized five species of large-spored trichophytons.

For two years Sabouraud was puzzled by the white downy growth on old cultures of trichophyton which he took to be contaminating moulds and not the irreversible change to sterility to which dermatophytes are prone and for which the term pleomorphism has also been applied (Fig. 12). Pleomorphism in dermatophytes has been much studied. Sabouraud devised his Conservation Agar, a 3% peptone medium containing no sugar, for the prevention of such change which is encouraged by sugar-containing media and delayed by culture on natural media such as wheat or barley grains.

The time was favourable for the reception of Sabouraud's findings which attracted world-wide interest and by the closing years of the century his evidence that there were many species of dermatophytes was generally accepted. The climax of this interest occurred at the Third International Congress of Dermatology held in London in 1896 when the afternoon of Thursday 6 August was devoted to 'Ringworm and the Trichophytons' – one of the most important sessions of the Congress according to the *British Journal of Dermatology*. The opening speaker was Dr Sabouraud, on 'Les trichophyties et la teigne tondant de Gruby', who dealt with special techniques, the plurality of the trichophytons, their general morphology, and ringworm caused by *Microsporum audouinii*. He also exhibited 300 cultures. He was followed by Professor A. J. Rosenbach of Göttingen, 'Über die Tiefen und eiternden Trichophyton-Erkrankungen und der Krankheitserreger', and Malcolm Morris (Fig. 10) of London whose contribution was the basis for his book, *Ringworm in the light of recent research*, 1898. Subsequent speakers included Charles J. White (Boston, USA), H. Leslie Roberts (Liverpool), H. G. Adamson, Colcott Fox and Frank Blaxall (London), and Professor P. G. Unna (Hamburg) (Fig. 10). In addition contributions were made, or taken as read, from France, Italy, and Spain. The text of the symposium occupied more than a hundred pages of the Official Proceedings (1898). Leslie Roberts protested that to separate *Microsporum audouinii* from the trichophyta would be 'an act of mutilation which would violate the principles of science and of common sense' but his was a lone voice. The plurality of the ringworm fungi was established.

Many of the common dermatomycoses and dermatophytes were first differentiated about this time. For example, in 1892 Djélaleddin-Moukhtar (a doctor of the Imperial Ottoman Army) was the first to publish on ringworm of the hands and feet, Bodin (1902) described *Trichophyton*

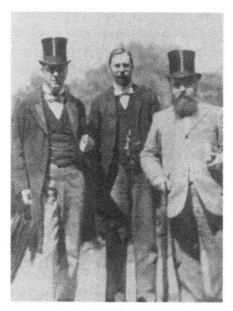

Fig. 10. Malcolm Morris (1847–1924) (left), Radcliffe Crocker (1845–1929) (centre), London dermatologists, and Prof. P. G. Unna (1850–1929) (right) of Vienna. *c*. 1896. (*Br.J.Derm.* **50**: 515, 1938).

violaceum, Castellani (1910) *T. rubrum* (as *Epidermophyton rubrum*) from Ceylon (Sri Lanka), and Sabouraud (1910) proposed the name *Epidermophyton inguinale* for the fungus (now *E. floccosum*) responsible for eczema marginatum (tinea cruris, ringworm of the groin) first clinically differentiated by Ferdinand von Hebra in 1860. Animal infections included ringworm of cattle (*T. verrucosum*; Bodin, 1902) and the horse (*T. equinum*; Gedoelst, 1902), fowl favus (*Microsporum gallinae,; as T. gallinae* by Mégnin, 1881) and the fungus causing cat and dog ringworm was named *M. canis* by Bodin (1902), *M. felineum* by Mewborn (1902), and *M. lanosum* by Sabouraud (1910) (see Chapter 3).

The taxonomic problem

The nutritive requirements of ringworm fungi are not exacting. Providing nitrogen is available in an organic form, such as that offered by the amino-acid mixture of a protein, most dermatophytes make profuse growth on a variety of media and in order that the results obtained by different workers might be correlated many attempts have been made to standardize diagnostic culture media. The most widely used has been the peptone-sugar medium known as 'Sabouraud's agar', which was the 'test medium' developed by Sabouraud (see above). Unfortunately Sabouraud used a particular French peptone, Granulée de Chassaing, which has not been generally available since the First World War, in combination with a special brand of impure maltose (Brute de Chanut) or glucose (Massée de Chanut). Later workers have substituted pure glucose or maltose and other types of peptone.

The importance of the composition of the medium is in part due to the emphasis Sabouraud and others placed on macrosopic characters such as whether the colony is cottony (floccose, lanose), powdery, or smooth (glabrous) and the patterns of the folds or convolution of the surface. Emphasis on these features was, unfortunately, aggravated by the fine series of photogravure plates illustrating cultural features which Sabouraud published in *Les teignes* (see Figs 11, 12). After the publication of that classic, medical men with little knowledge of mycology tended to make their identifications by matching cultures against Sabouraud's figures without any attempt to ascertain the characters of the spores and other microscopical features which Sabouraud ' knew were of great taxonomic importance.

Dermatophytes produce three types of asexual spores in culture: large *macroconidia* (the 'fuseaux' and 'spindles' of French and British dermatologists, respectively), small unicellular, globular, or pear-shaped *microconidia*, and thick-walled resting *chlamydospores* (see Fig. 14). Macroconidia are usually produced in smaller numbers than microconidia. They are generally most readily produced in a 'primary' culture (the culture derived from an inoculum of infected material) and sometimes, as in *Microsporum audouinii* and *Trichophyton violaceum*, it is the lack of the appropriate growth substances which prevents their development (Hazen, 1947; Georg, 1949). Among other microscopic structures are the hyphae composed of cells each dilated at one end, the so-called 'racquette hyphae', *spiral hyphae* (hyphae coiled like springs), and 'nodular organs' which are possibly vestigial ascogonia.

When classifying parasitic micro-organisms the systematist must always decide on the importance, if any, of host–parasitic relationships as taxonomic criteria and much confusion in the classification of the ringworm fungi resulted in the failure of different workers to agree on the importance to be attached to clinical as opposed to mycological characters. Sabouraud, as a medical man and experienced clinician, favoured clinical characters for the delimitation of genera. The four genera which he recog-

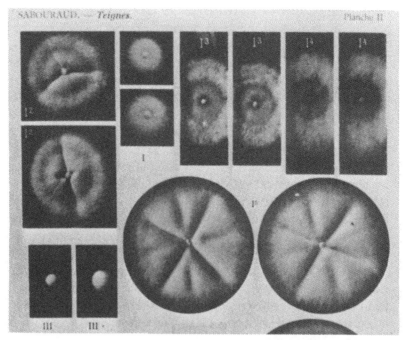

Fig. 11. *Microsporum audouinii* cultures. (Sabouraud, 1910, part of plate ii).

nized in *Les teignes* were distinguished by the type of lesion and the spatial relationship of the fungus to the infected hair. Species of *Epidermophyton* attached skin but not hair. The genus *Achorion* was reserved for fungi giving rise to the scutula characteristic of clinical favus. *Microsporum* was differentiated by the mosaic-like sheath of small spores around the hair shaft from *Trichophyton* in which the spores were arranged in linear series. The genus *Trichophyton* was subdivided into two series according to whether the fungus developed on the surface of the hair (*Ectothrix*) or within the hair (*Endothrix*). Twenty years later Sabouraud revised this classification and, while still maintaining the importance of clinical criteria, replaced *Trichophyton* by *Endothrix*, *Microides*, and *Megaspore* (Sabouraud, 1929), three genera which have been little used (see Table 1).

Grigoraki may be noticed as an author who took up an extreme mycological position and devised an elaborate classification, based on macroscopic and microscopic cultural characters necessitating the creation of six new genera (Grigoraki, 1925, 1929; Guiart & Grigoraki, 1928). The French mycologist Vuillemin (1931) distributed a number of the ringworm

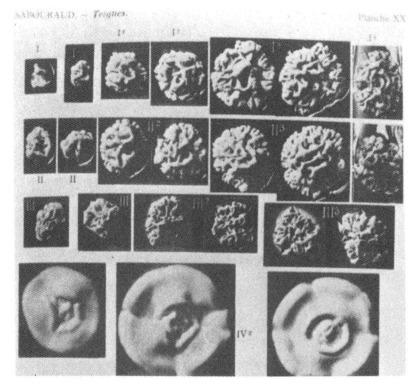

Fig. 12. *Trichophyton schoenleinii* cultures. Bottom row, pleomorphic state. (Sabouraud, 1910, part of plate xx.)

fungi among 'non-medical' genera of the Fungi Imperfecti and the American C. W. Dodge (1935) employed eight genera and numerous subgenera in the primarily mycological classification he devised.

There is a general agreement among mycologists today that genera of fungi are best delimited on morphological grounds and a most important advance in the classification of dermatophytes was the demonstration by the American C. W. Emmons (Fig. 13), the first mycologist by training to be employed by the United States Department of Health, that three of Sabouraud's genera could be satisfactorily defined in mycological terms (Emmons, 1934).[11] In Emmons' scheme the most important diagnostic criterion was the character of the macroconidium. In the genus *Microsporum* the macroconidium is more or less spindle-shaped, multiseptate, and thick-walled; club-shaped, multiseptate, and thin-walled in *Trichophyton*; pear-shaped, with no, or only a few septa in *Epidermophyton* (Fig. 14). Other characters which served to differentiate these three genera were

Table 1. *Generic classifications of the dermatophytes*

Sabouraud (1910)	Sabouraud (1929)	Emmons (1934)	Langeron (*Précis*, 1945)
[a]*Microsporum* Gruby, 1843 (Type: *M. audouinii* Gruby)	*Microsporum* Gruby	*Microsporum* Gruby	*Sabouraudites* Ota & Langeron, 1923 (Type: *S. audouinii* (Gruby) Ota & Langeron)
[b]*Trichophyton* Malmsten, 1845 (Type: *T. tonsurans* Malmsten) with two series:		*Trichophyton* Malmsten	*Trichophyton* Malmsten with two subgenera
Endothrix	*Endothrix* Sabouraud, 1929		*Endotrichophyton* Langeron *Favotrichophyton* (Neveu-Lemaire) Langeron *Ctenomyces* Eidam, 1880 (Type: *C. serratus* Eidam)
Ectothrix	*Microides* Sabouraud, 1929 *Megaspore* Sabouraud, 1929		
Epidermophyton Sabouraud, 1910 (Type: *E. inguinale* (Sabouraud, 1907) Sabouraud)	*Epidermophyton* Sabouraud	*Epidermophyton* Sabouraud	*Epidermophyton* Sabouraud
Achorion Remak, 1845 (Type: *A. schoenleinii* (Lebert, 1845) Remak)			

[a] Teleomorph *Nannizzia* Stockdale, 1961; [b] Teleomorph *Arthroderma* Currey, 1860; [c] No teleomorph known. *No type specified.

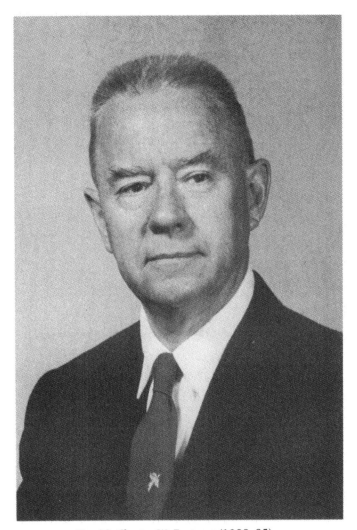

Fig. 13. Chester W. Emmons (1900–85).

shown to be correlated with macroconidial characters. The species which Sabouraud included in the genus *Achorion* were found to be naturally accommodated in *Microsporum* or *Trichophyton* as delimited by Emmons and *Epidermophyton* was reduced to a monotypic genus for *E. floccosum* (syn. *E. inguinale*).

The generic proposals of Emmons are those on which the current taxonomy of the dermatophytes is based. Medical mycologists of the French school, however, frequently followed the classification developed

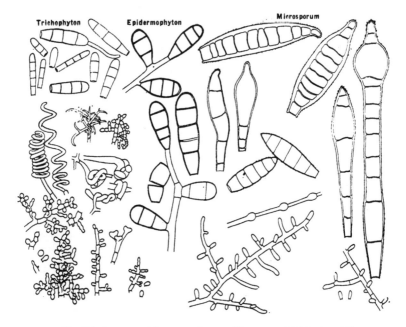

Fig. 14. Genera of dermatophytes. (Emmons, 1934, Fig. 27).

by Professor Langeron, two of whose generic uses call for comment. Langeron & Milochevitch (1930) interpreted the conidial masses associated with branched antler-like hyphae exhibited by certain species of *Trichophyton* as perithecia and considered that it would make for a more 'natural' classification if these species were classified, not as Fungi Imperfecti but as Ascomycetes, that is as 'perfect fungi', and it was to the genus *Ctenomyces* of the family Gymnoascaceae that Langeron and Milochevitch transferred these species. Langeron's other innovation was to widen the genus *Microsporum*, as a new genus *Sabouraudites*, to include certain species of *Trichophyton* (Ota & Langeron, 1923) (see Table 1).

In 1899 Matruchot and Dassonville concluded that dermatophytes were asexual ('imperfect' or anamorphic) states of ascomycetes possibly related to the Gymnoascaceae. The first sexual ('perfect' or teleomorphic) state of a dermatophyte to be reported was the ascigerous state of *Microsporum gypseum*, named *Gymnoascus gypseus*, by the Italian mycologist Arturo Nannizzi of Siena in 1927 (Fig. 15). This claim was widely discredited for the next thirty years until Griffin (1960) in Australia rediscovered *G. gypseus* and Phyllis Stockdale (1961), at the Commonwealth Mycological Institute, Kew, independently described the perfect state of another member

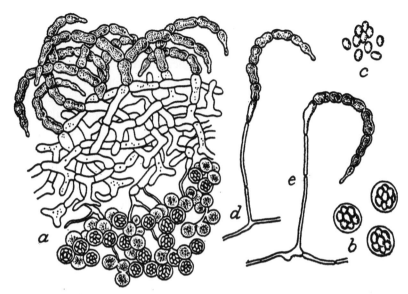

Fig. 15. *Gymnoascus gypseus* Nannizzi, teleomorphic ('perfect') state of *Microsporum gypseum*. (Nannizzi, 1927).

of the *Microsporum gypseum* group for which she proposed the new genus *Nannizzia*. Simultaneously, J. C. Gentles and Christine Dawson, working in Glasgow, described and named teleomorphic states of two geophyllic trichophytons and of *M. nanum* (Dawson & Gentles, 1959, 1961). Many more teleomorphic states have since been described and many dermatophytes shown to be heterothallic, two cultures of appropriate mating type having to undergo fusion for ascocarp production to be achieved.

Variation

Sabouraud, as is usual for any taxonomist approaching a new group for the first time, drew his species concept too narrowly. He did not take the range of variation within the species on which there have been many investigations into account. The studies by Emmons on spontaneous variation in *Microsporum gypseum* and *Trichophyton mentagrophytes* indicated the very wide differences between variants produced from one single-spore culture. Later Emmons & Hollaender (1945) produced a bewildering number of variants in *T. mentagrophytes* by the experimental irradiation of spores with ultraviolet light while Mackinnon & Artagaveytia-Allende (1948) first showed physiological differences in respect of vitamin requirements between strains within the species

T. discoides and *T. ochraceum*. Nutritional requirements were also investigated in the United States by Rhoda Benham (1948, 1953), Lucille Georg (1950, 1952) and Margarita Silva & Benham (1952) and exploited by the development of nutritionally based identification tests.

The description of dermatophytes by strictly mycological criteria, combined with the discovery that some occur naturally in the soil where they are related to a series of similar fungi (see Chapter 5), exploded the myth that they belong to a special group of 'medical fungi' – and similar conclusions apply to the other fungi pathogenic for man and animals. For dermatophytes this has meant that the hundreds of species, and the more than a thousand names applied to them, found scattered through the literature, have been reduced to less than fifty which greatly simplifies the position and greatly reduces misunderstanding between different investigators, whether clinicians or mycologists. Outstanding problems of course remain, as for example, that common to all students of pathogenic micro-organisms, how best to taxonomize host specialization and virulence.

3

Names: problems of nomenclature

Having delimited the mycoses and the pathogens, the problems of giving them unambiguous names remained. The ideal, that each disease and each pathogen should each have one name, is unattainable. Since Latin ceased to be the *lingua franca* common names for diseases have been in the vernacular and so vary from one language to another while the nomenclature of the pathogens must allow taxonomists who differ in their opinions on how a pathogen should be classified to be able to reflect this difference in their nomenclature.

During the second half of the nineteenth century the need to regulate the use of the scientific names applied to living organisms became increasingly apparent. Botanists were the first to respond with the *Lois de la nomenclature botanique* as adopted by the International Botanical Congress held in Paris in 1867. In 1901 zoologists followed with a very similar, but independent, Code as adopted by the Fifth International Congress of Zoology. Thus one name for any taxon of given circumscription was assured and the duplication of identical names within the plant or animal kingdoms avoided but this did not prevent one generic name being accepted by both Codes – for example, *Drosophila* is applied to both a genus of fruit-flies and a genus of larger fungi (toadstools). The *International Code of Botanical Nomenclature* regulates most aspects of nomenclatural procedure and has been revised most frequently. The current Code is the 13th edition as adopted by the Sydney International Botanical Congress of 1981. The corresponding Zoological Code of 1985 is essentially the 3rd edition.

Applied biologists continually complain about the name changes instituted by taxonomists but during the last fifty years they have increasingly realized the difference between international nomenclature which is obligatory and taxonomy which is a matter of judgement (to which response need not always be hurried) and the greater stability in nomenclature obtained by using names in line with the Codes.

The scientific names of fungi are subject to the International Botanical

33

Code (those of actinomycetes to the essentially similar International Code of Nomenclature of Bacteria and Viruses) which specifies the conditions for the form, publication, and selection of the correct name for any particular taxonomic circumscription. The starting point for the nomenclature of fungi is 1753, the date of publication of Linnaeus, *Species plantarum*, which includes a few fungus names, but bacteriologists recently adopted 1980 as the starting point for bacterial names.

In general the correct name for any organism is the earliest (first) name published in line with the requirements of the Code of Nomenclature. For example, the cat and dog ringworm fungus has been widely known under three binomials which satisfy the Code: *Microsporum canis* Bodin (1902), *M. felineum* Mewborn (1902), and *M. lanosum* Sabouraud (1910). The correct name is *M. canis* which antedates *M. felineum* because Mewborn in his paper mentions Bodin's book published earlier in the same year. The appropriateness of names cannot be taken into account. The cat may be more frequently infected than the dog but two names can be used only if it is considered that the Microsporum ringworm of the cat and dog are caused by different species.

The aim of the Botanical Code is, according to the Preamble, 'the provision of a stable method of naming taxonomic groups, avoiding and rejecting the use of names which may cause error or ambiguity or throw science into confusion'. To avoid confusion the Code allows certain exceptions to the Rules. The most significant of these is when an earlier generic name has been overlooked, a later name is in general use, and a reversion to the earlier name would cause much confusion. An International Botanical congress may then sanction the 'conservation' of the later name against the earlier. For example, the Congress of 1954 conserved the generic name *Candida* Berkhout (1923) against the earlier *Syringospora* Quinquaud (1868) (see Chapter 4) because of the confusion that would have resulted from changing names such as *C. albicans* which are in daily use.

Although the International Botanical Code was designed for plants, there are a number of special provisions for mycologists. Notably among these are those relating to the nomenclature of the teleomorphic ('perfect', sexual) and anamorphic ('imperfect', asexual) states of fungi. Briefly, the name of the *teleomorph* takes precedence and covers both states but any name given to an *anamorph* may be used as appropriate. For example, *Nannizzia gypseum* takes precedence over *Microsporum gypseum* although the latter is the one normally in use in the diagnostic laboratory where the teleomorph of this species is rarely seen. At times both anamorphic and teleomorphic states of one species have been described and named as distinct taxa without the connexion between them being recognized. In 1911 the famous Italian taxonomic mycologist, P.A. Saccardo described and named the anamorphic fungus isolated from an Italian case of white grain mycetoma as *Monosporium apiospermum*. In 1922 C. L. Shear in the United States described and named the teleomorphic – ascospore-producing – isolate from mycetoma of the foot in Texas as *Allescheria boydii* (in honour of the physician attending the case). It was twenty-two years later that Emmons (1944) showed the two fungi to be states of one fungus when he obtained the ascosporic state of *M. apiospermum* from a Canadian case of mycetoma. Because of changes in taxonomic opinion and the application of the rules of nomenclature the names of both states have recently undergone changes. The Canadian mycologist W. S. Malloch considered that the teleomorph did not belong to the genus *Allescheria* Saccardo & Sydow, 1899, and so transferred it to a new genus *Petriellidium* Malloch, 1970, for which the earlier valid name *Pseudallescheria* Negroni & Fischer, 1943, had to be substituted – hence *Pseudallescheria boydii* (Shear, 1922) McGinnis, Padhye & Ajello, 1982 – while the genus *Monosporium* Bonorden, 1851, is now considered to be illegitimate under the Code so that the current correct name for the anamorph is *Scedosporium apiospermum* (Saccardo, 1911) Castellani & Chalmers, 1919. A generalization from such complications is that any worker using a scientific name for a pathogen in line with the relevant Code enhances his position to promote the use of the same name by others.

Disease nomenclature

Disease names are not subject to strict international control. Their usage tends to reflect local practice. Clinicians have coined many relatively unspecific disease names for fungal infections by qualifying the suffix '-mycosis' according to the part of the body affected; e.g. bronchomycosis, dermatomycosis, otomycosis, etc. Another popular method has been to derive disease names from generic names of the pathogens; e.g. aspergillosis, sporotrichosis, microsporosis, trichophytosis, etc., and it has often been felt necessary to change the disease name in line with taxonomic changes in the circumscription of the pathogen. For example, 'moniliasis', which for long had universal currency and could have been retained as a name with interesting historical overtones, has become 'candidosis' while white grain mycetoma during recent years has been variously designated 'allescheriasis', 'monosporiosis', 'petriellidiosis', and 'pseudallescheriasis' to match the changing taxonomy of the pathogen. Some at one time universally used latinized names but of indefinite circumscription have either fallen out of use (e.g. porrigo) or have survived with a precise application, as has 'herpes' which, once commonly applied to ringworm, is in current usage restricted to certain viral infections.

Plant pathologists had earlier experienced the same problems and in 1928 the Plant Pathology Committee of the British Mycological Society published a *List of common names of British plant diseases* in an attempt to increase uniformity in disease nomenclature. This was only partially successful but a more successful outcome was an increase in uniformity in the nomenclature of the pathogens, the names of which were in line with the International Code of Botanical Nomenclature. Further editions were called for and in 1939 no less than 42 'Offices, Societies and Institutes' in the United Kingdom agreed to 'respect the recommended names for fungi as closely as possible in their official publications'. In 1946 The Medical Research Council's Medical Mycology Committee[1] (which included four mycologists who had served on the BMS Plant Pathology Committee) initiated a similar list which was first published in January 1950 as *MRC Memorandum 23*, 'Nomenclature of fungi pathogenic to man and animals. Names recommended for use in Great Britain'. This list was widely distributed (revised editions appearing in 1958, 1967, 1977) and it did much to promote uniformity in nomenclatural practice while serving as an example to others. At the Fifth International Microbiological Congress in Brazil, 1950, the Special Committee on Medical and Veterinary Mycopathology (which had been set up in 1948 after the Fourth Congress) drew up the first international list of recommended names of fungi pathogenic for man and animals (Nickerson, 1952) while the Royal College of Physicians when preparing the 8th and final edition of *Nomenclature of Diseases* published in 1960 included, for the first time, a mycologist among the compilers. Later there were similar but more comprehensive listings of both mycoses and their causal agents, e.g. in the *International Nomenclature of Diseases*, a joint product of the World Health Organization (WHO) and the Council for International Organizations of Medical Science (CIOMS).[2]

The 1950 International Congress for Microbiology was the first international congress to include a Section on Mycology – convened by A. E. de Arêa Lêao of the Instituto Oswaldo Cruz, Rio de Janeiro – restricted to medical and veterinary mycology. As a result a group of mycopathologists from North and South America and Europe, all staying in the same hotel at Petropolis, situated in the mountains some 40 miles from Rio, spent a

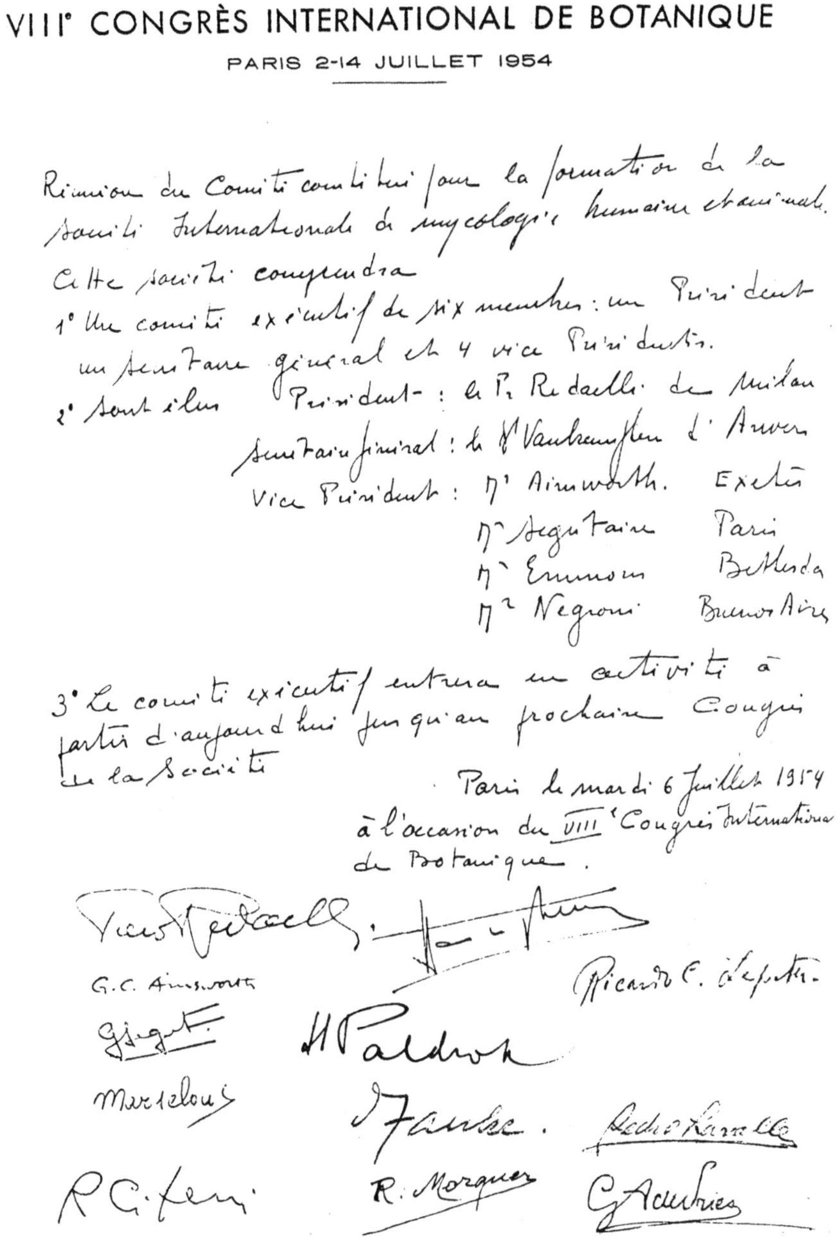

VIIIe CONGRÈS INTERNATIONAL DE BOTANIQUE

PARIS 2-14 JUILLET 1954

Réunion du Comité constitué pour la formation de la Société Internationale de mycologie humaine et animale.

Cette société comprendra

1° Un comité exécutif de six membres: un Président un Secrétaire général et 4 vice Présidents.

2° Sont élus Président: le Pr Redaelli de Milan

Secrétaire général: le Dr Vanbreuseghem d'Anvers

Vice Président: Mr Ainsworth. Exeter

Mr Segretain Paris

Mr Emmons Bethesda

Mr Negroni Buenos Aires

3° Le comité exécutif entrera en activité à partir d'aujourd'hui jusqu'au prochain Congrès de la Société

Paris le mardi 6 Juillet 1954

à l'occasion du VIII Congrès International de Botanique.

G.C. Ainsworth

Fig. 16. Foundation document of the International Society for Human and Animal Mycology (ISHAM).

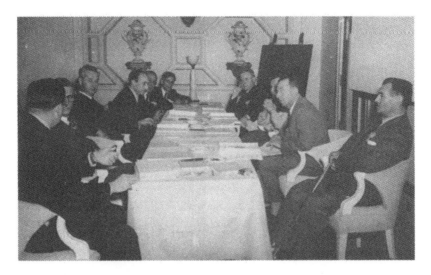

Fig. 17. The Special Committee on Medical and Veterinary Mycopathology in session at the Fifth International Congress for Microbiology, Rio de Janeiro, August 1950.

(Left to right) J. W. Nickerson (USA), A. L. Carrión (Puerto Rico), F. de Almeida (Brazil), P. Negroni (Argentina), A. C. Arêa Leão (Brazil), G. Segretain (France), C. W. Emmons (USA), G. C. Ainsworth (UK), J. E. Mackinnon (Uruguay), P. Redaelli (Italy).

week of intense formal and informal wide-ranging discussions which among other things contributed to the decision of mycopathologists at the Sixth Congress, in Rome, in 1953, to set up an international mycopathological society. This decision was implemented at the International Botanical Congress in Paris, 1953, when the International Society for Human and Animal Mycology (ISHAM) was inaugurated (Fig. 16) with Professor Redaelli of Milan as president (Fig. 17) and Professor Vanbreuseghem of Antwerp as Secretary[3] (Fig. 56). ISHAM (to which, by 1985, 17 national mycopathological societies had affiliated) in 1961 founded the journal *Sabouraudia* (re-named *Journal of Medical and Veterinary Mycology* in 1986) and among its later activities was the compilation of an international English/French list of mycoses and the causal fungi.[4]

4

Problems of pathogenic status with special reference to mycelial yeasts

Questions of pathogenic status for long presented difficulties, as they still do. Early in the nineteenth century before the concept of pathogenicity had been established the English dermatologist Thomas Bateman [1778–1821] held the view that ringworm of the scalp seemed 'to originate spontaneously in children of feeble and flabby habits, or in a state approaching marasmus, who are ill fed, uncleanly, and not sufficiently exercised' (Bateman, 1813:169). That is to say he believed the disease to be constitutional, Samuel Plumbe [?–1837], the author of the popular *Practical treatise on diseases of the skin...*, 1824, thought otherwise, although he believed the constitution to be a major factor in favus. From his own observations and experiments, Plumbe confirmed the views of others that ringworm of the scalp and favus were contagious. He was the first to recognize the connexion between head and body ringworm, and his recommendations for treatment were enlightened. But the views expressed by Bateman were difficult to eradicate. In the fourth edition of his *Treatise*, published in 1837 after Bateman's death, Plumbe still thought it necessary to refute with vigour the suggestion that the occurrence of ringworm in several children of one school or family should be attributed 'to the season or some other common cause' (Bateman, 1813:231). The elucidation of the aetiology of ringworm by David Gruby during 1841–4 (as recounted in Chapter 2) was given a mixed reception. In France, A. P. E. Bazin advocated the acceptance of the parasitic origin of ringworm but in 1850 Alphée Cazenave was warning against 'the illusion of micrography' and denying the presence of 'any pathogenic properties in the mysterious atoms' of *Achorion schoenleinii*, the only fungus which he recognized (Morris, 1898). In Great Britain likewise opinion was divided. Bennett confirmed Gruby's results on favus experimentally (see Chapter 2). Sir William Jenner [1815–98], of smallpox vaccination fame, adopted the parasitic view of skin infection and thought that the simple way to effect a cure was to destroy the fungus by some topical application. 'But the error soon betrayed itself to his mind and he candidly acknowledged that this mode of treatment ended in disappointment' according to Jabez Hogg [1817–99], a constitutional diehard, who in 1873 reprinted in book form a series of papers published some years earlier fulminating against the parasitic theory of disease or, when the involvement of fungi in skin disease became indisputable, advocating the view that variations in these diseases were due to differences in constitution modifying the soil for one essential fungus (Hogg, 1873). At about the same time Erasmus Wilson [1809–84], the famous London dermatologist who paid for the transport of Cleopatra's Needle from Egypt to England and encouraged the daily bath, offered to leave his fortune to his young assistant Malcolm Morris [1847–1924] (Fig. 10) on condition the latter brought out a new edition of Wilson's *Treatise on diseases of the skin* (first issued in 1842) and in so doing should oppose unreservedly the doctrine of a parasitic causation of ringworm. After twenty-four hours consideration Morris declined the offer.[1] Wilson left his wealth elsewhere.

The mycotic origin of ringworm provided inspiration for the claim that fungi were also responsible for other diseases, particularly Asiatic cholera, a pandemic of which began in 1846 and spread to Europe. In 1849 a group of three Bristol doctors associated certain microscopic bodies which they interpreted as fungi with the aetiology of cholera but this conclusion was discredited by an investigation instigated by the Royal College of Physicians.[2] It was Professor Ernst Hallier of Jena who made the most spectacular claims in which by an experimental cultural procedure which did not prevent contamination (see Bulloch (1938):189–92) he associated not only cholera (produced, he claimed, by *Urocystis*, a smut fungus of rice in India) but also variola (smallpox), vaccinia (cowpox), measles, typhoid, and typhus each with a particular species of mould. These findings, which were widely publicised in the popular press, were warned against by the Rev. M. J. Berkeley in his presidential address to Section D (Biology) of the British Association meeting at Norwich in 1868.[3]

Following the introduction of techniques for growing bacteria and fungi in pure culture and the determination of the correct relationship of a fungus (or other agent) to a disease by the application of the so-called 'Koch's Postulates' ((1) establishing that the organism is regularly associated with the disease; (2) isolating the organism in pure culture; and (3) showing that the isolate is capable of producing the disease) questions of pathogenic status such as those considered above are easily resolved without controversy. However there are other situations in which the pathogenic status is not so easily established when both clinical and mycological findings have to be critically assessed before a decision can be reached. Such cases frequently involve pathogenic yeasts (particularly mycelial yeasts of the genus *Candida*) which are often found associated with apparently normal individuals and which for mycopathological interest (as judged by the size of the literature) have only been surpassed by the dermatophytes.

Yeast infections

'Yeast' has no precise mycological meaning. In popular usage it is applied to unicellular fungi which multiply by budding but the term also covers forms which reproduce by fission and yeasts (often distinguished as 'mycelial yeasts') regularly associated with mycelium or pseudomycelium, the hyphal-like elements of the latter being interpreted as elongated buds. (The yeast-like phases produced under special circumstances by normally mycelial fungi, especially those discussed under dimorphism in Chapter 5, are, however, usually excluded from the group by yeast taxonomists.)

Yeasts in general may be divided into two major series: *sporogenous yeasts*, such as bakers' or brewers' yeast (*Saccharomyces cerevisiae*), which have a teleomorphic (sexual) phase and *asporogenous yeasts*, which are anamorphic (asexual). Most yeasts pathogenic for man and animals belong to the second category or are treated as being anamorphic. Because the ability to ferment sugary solutions is a general character of most yeasts and because of the paucity of morphological features available as taxonomic criteria, fermentative ability and other biochemical features have always been given prominence in yeast taxonomy. For example, Berg in 1846 performed biochemical experiments with the thrush fungus which demonstrated the ability of scabs of aphthae to coagulate human and cow's milk in six to 24 hours and he also compared the results of the addition of the thrush fungus or bakers' yeast to solutions of cane and milk sugars, noting the reaction 24 hours later. With the rise of bacteriology where biochemical tests are standard practice for differentiating species, similar tests were systematically developed for characterizing yeasts. Many new species of yeasts associated with disorders in man and animals were proposed and, as for dermatophytes (see Chapter 2), yeast taxonomy and nomenclature became chaotic. This situation was finally rectified largely by a group of workers associated with the special yeast collection of the Dutch Centraalbureau voor Schimmelcultures maintained at the Technical High School at Delft from where a series of authoritative monographs emanated and influenced yeast studies throughout the world. Particularly notable was Lodder and Krieger-van Rij's monograph of 1952, revised editions of which appeared in 1970 and 1984.

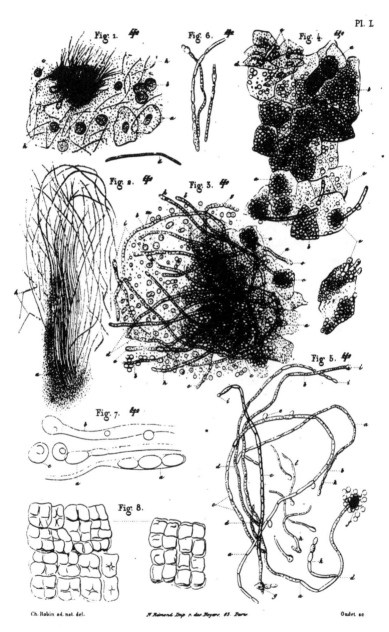

Fig. 1 et 2. Algue de la bouche. Fig. 3 à-7. Champignon du Muguet. F. 8. Sarcina.

Fig. 18. *Candida albicans* (Figs 3–7). (Robin, 1853, plate i).

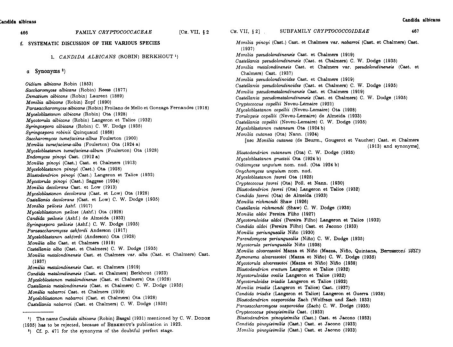

Fig. 19. Partial synonymy of *Candida albicans*. (Lodder & Krieger-van Rij, 1952: 466–7).

Candidosis[4]

The most important yeasts pathogenic for man (and higher animals) are a group related to the thrush fungus which has a chequered nomenclatural history. Described but not named by Langenbeck (1839), Berg (1841), and Gruby (1842a), the thrush fungus was first designated *Oidium albicans* by Robin (1853) (Fig. 18) In 1868 Quinquaud[5] proposed a new genus *Syringospora* to accommodate the thrush fungus as *S. robinii* while from 1890 Zopf's error in transferring Robin's taxon to the genus *Monilia*[6] was widely followed and this gave rise to 'moniliasis' as the disease name. In 1923 Christine Berkhout of Delft clarified the position by proposing a new genus *Candida* with *C. albicans* as the type and as noted in Chapter 3 her generic name was subsequently conserved against the earlier *Syringospora*. The genus *Candida* has a worldwide distribution and the thrush fungus has been described under many names – Lodder & Krieger-van Rij (1952) listed 87 synonyms distributed through a dozen genera (see Fig. 19).

Both before and after the 1914–18 war the study of medical yeasts was dominated by Professor Marchese Sir Aldo Castellani (Fig. 20), a

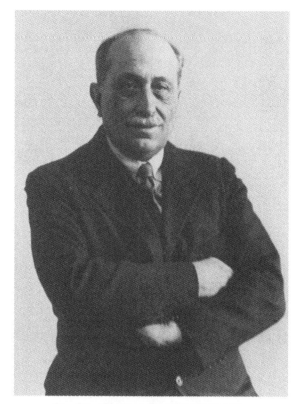

Fig. 20. Aldo Castellani (1877–1971).

remarkable man. Born and educated in Florence, Castellani then studied under Professor Walther Kruse [1864–1943] in Bonn and (in 1901) Patrick Manson at the London School of Tropical Medicine. The next year, as a member of the Royal Society's Commission to Uganda on Sleeping Sickness, he proved that this disease is caused by a trypanosome. From 1903 Castellani was bacteriologist to the Ceylon [Sri Lanka] government and in 1906 elucidated the aetiology of yaws. In 1915 he returned to Europe and by the end of the First World War was at the same time Lieutenant Colonel in the Royal Italian Medical Service and Admiral in the corresponding branch of the navy. Next, successively (or sometimes concurrently), he was consultant to the Ministry of Pensions in London, on the staff of the Ross Institute, lecturer on mycology at the London School of Hygiene & Tropical Medicine, and professor of tropical medicine at Tulane University, New Orleans. In addition he built up a Harley Street practice of unprecedented proportions with many royal and aristocratic patients. (On one occasion, it is said, he had three European queens in his consulting rooms at the same time.) He was called to Italy as a physician to attend Mussolini and during the Italo-Ethiopian war became Surgeon-General to the Italian Forces. On the entry of Italy into the Second World War, Castellani sought refuge in the Italian embassy and returned to Italy under diplomatic immunity. (His culture collection had to be left behind but it survived the war due to the dedication of his loyal technician, Mr D. Press.) After the war he lived in Portugal where he was medical adviser to the exiled Italian Royal family, wrote a flamboyant autobiography (*Microbes, man, and monarchs*, 1960), and continued with microbiological studies.

Castellani was a prolific writer – the author of some two hundred publications on medical mycology alone. Many of these are of indifferent quality. Few are now cited and most of the many new names he introduced are in synonymy. The *Manual of tropical medicine*, 1910, written in collaboration with A. J. Chalmers, was much used, particularly the bulky third edition of 1919, and Castellani's colourful personality, enthusiasm, and generosity did much to promote medical mycology in the United Kingdom and elsewhere during the interwar years. He was, however, an able and acute observer and was the first to recognize *Trichophyton rubrum* and, among yeasts, *Candida tropicalis* (1910), *C. krusei* (1910), *C. pseudo-tropicalis* (1911), and *C. guilliermondii* (1912), all well known worldwide today.

Species of Candida are differentiated according to their abilities to ferment or assimilate a range of sugars and other compounds, the assimilation tests commonly being made by the auxanogramic method.[7] Tests for ascertaining whether the yeast is mycelial have been developed (e.g. incubation overnight in a starch water medium) and two special tests that have been developed for distinguishing *C. albicans* are: (1) incubation of cells in serum for 3 hours at 37 °C when only those of *C. albicans* produce hyphae (Taschdjian *et al.*, 1960); (2) inoculation of corn meal agar (see Benham, 1931) or other solid medium when spherical, thick-walled chlamydospores develop terminally on the pseudomycelium when the result is positive. Castellani (1937) by using thirteen carbohydrates and other special tests recognized more than thirty species of *Monilia* [*Candida*] of medical importance in contrast to the half-dozen accepted today which may be distinguished by the fermentation of four sugars (glucose, maltose, sucrose, lactose).

There have been a number of investigations, particularly in Japan, on applications of the antigenic structure of Candida and other yeasts to their taxonomy and identification but achievements have been limited because of the many antigenic components that related yeasts have in common. One finding that has been widely confirmed is that of Hasenclever who was the first to establish two antigenic groups, A and B, among strains of *Candida albicans* (see Hasenclever & Mitchell, 1961–3).

The expression of candidosis is remarkable for its diversity. With the exception of the hair, virtually no part of the human body is immune from infection which may occur at any time from the prenatal and neonatal periods to terminal illness in old age. The classical location for candidosis is the mouth, especially of infants (but denture stomatitis associated with Candida in the elderly has a higher incidence) while other infections of the oral region include angular cheilitis (perlèche), candida leukoplakia, candida glossitis, infection of the tonsils, and dental caries. Interdigital candidosis (erosio interdigitalis blastomycetica) may be confused with ringworm and though glabrous skin is rarely affected chronic granulomatous lesions may develop at mucocutaneous sites. Onychia and paronychia are not uncommon. Candidosis of the external ear has been reported and sterile candidids (see Chapter 5) may arise on the skin as an allergic response to infection. The genitalia are affected. Candida balanitis, balanoposthitis, and urethritis in the male are usually contracted, like neonatal thrush, from vulvo-vaginal infection of the female, an infection of common occurrence on which there is a very extensive literature. Both the gastro-intestinal tract (particularly the oesophagus) and the respiratory system may be involved. Renal candidosis has been reported (together with candida cystitis and urethritis) as have infections of the spleen, brain (and other parts of the central nervous system), biliary tract, heart (endocarditis), bones and joints, and the eye (including the lacrimal apparatus). Candida peritonitis is on record, as is disseminated candidosis (candida septicaemia) when the pathogen may be isolated from the blood. Finally, injection abscesses caused by *C. albicans* may be mentioned.[8] Candidosis in animals is of less importance. Avian candidosis in young chickens, turkeys, and geese involving infection of the crop occurs (see Blaxland & Fincham, 1950) and Candida has been associated with bovine mastitis and mycotic abortion.[9]

Although candidosis is contagious infections not infrequently originate endogenously. Rarely isolated from human skin, Candida is often present in the oropharangeal region (especially in the mouths of those wearing dentures; Knighton, 1939) and faeces of normal individuals and the vagina of women, especially pregnant women, showing no signs of vaginitis. The attribution of a causal relationship of Candida to an associated pathological condition has thus often to be made with caution.

During the nineteen-twenties it was thought that *Candida albicans* (as *Monilia albicans*) played an important part in the aetiology of tropical sprue since the fungus was frequently found in the stools of affected persons. Later work led to the conclusion that sprue was due to a nutritional deficiency and that Candida infection was a secondary effect. Candidosis of the respiratory tract has been a long-standing diagnostic problem since the clinical account by Rosén von Rosenstein in 1771 and the case of pulmonary mycosis described by Bennett (1844). The modern era originated with Castellani's description in 1905 of 'pulmonary moniliasis' or 'tea taster's cough' which he found to be an occupational disease of tea tasters in Sri Lanka (Castellani, 1927–8). Tea taster's cough is an allergic response to the inhalation of yeasts and other particles when samples of tea are tested for their aroma before infusion. Castellani associated the condition with several species of *Candida* (*Monilia* in his terminology). Subsequently records of pulmonary candidosis were reported from many parts of the world although in the United Kingdom workers inclined to the view that the presence of Candida in these cases was usually incidental and in 1936 J. F. D. Shrewsbury of Birmingham University Medical School in the light of extensive examination of the occurrence of Candida in tuberculosis sputum and in oral, nasal, and throat swabs from healthy babies and adults came to the conclusion that 'A critical review of the literature of bronchomoniliasis does not reveal any convincing reasons for the retention of the name in medical nosology'. Twenty years later Riddel & Clayton (1958) of the Brompton Hospital, on clinical, serological, and radiological evidence firmly endorsed this conclusion although they granted that there are rare cases of primary pulmonary candidiosis. Candida does cause secondary thrush of the bronchi.

Aspergillosis

Aspergillosis in animals and man includes a number of well defined pathological conditions. Avian aspergillosis of the lungs and air-sacs has been recognized for two centuries (see Chapter 1). It was Fresenius in 1863 who introduced the term aspergillosis when investigating the infection of the air-sacs of a bustard (*Otis tarda*) by the mould he described as *Aspergillus fumigatus* (Fresenius, 1850–63:81) (Fig. 21) while human pulmonary aspergillosis, probably first reported by Sluyter (1847), was accurately described by Virchow (1856) in a paper which is now a classic (Fig. 21). Cohnheim (1865) described two more similar cases, Ernst (1894) infection of the kidney, and in 1897 the French veterinarian Adrien Lucet

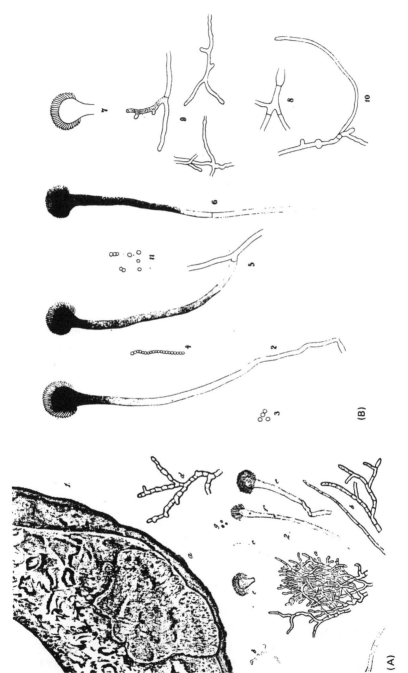

Fig. 21. A. Pulmonary aspergillosis in man. 1, part of lung showing lesion; 2, *Aspergillus [fumigatus]*. (Virchow, 1856, part of plate iv.) B. *Aspergillus fumigatus* Fresenius. 2, from lungs and air sacs of a bustard; 4–11, from human lung. (Fresenius, 1850–63, part of plate x).

[1858–1916] and Louis Rénon, professor of medical pathology in Paris, independently monographed aspergillosis in animals and animals and man.

Aspergillosis is caused by several species of *Aspergillus* including *A. flavus*, *A. nidulans*, *A. niger*, and *A. terreus* but principally *A. fumigatus*. Most isolates of *A. fumigatus*, which over the years has probably been more often correctly identified than most fungi responsible for mycotic infection in man and animals, are pathogenic but the significance of its association with a pathological condition has, like that of *Candida* but for different reasons, often to be assessed with caution. It is ubiquitous on vegetable residues, has unspecialized nutritional requirements, and grows well at 37 °C (the temperature routinely used for incubating cultures of bacterial pathogens). In addition the spores are readily airborne, small (2.5–3.0 μm diam.) and so able to penetrate deeply into the respiratory system; thus *A. fumigatus* is a not uncommon contaminant of cultures and sputum, etc.

Aspergilli, especially *Aspergillus niger*, have frequently been associated with infection of the external ear, usually, according to some,[10] associated with primary bacterial infection, but evidence of mycotic otitis caused by aspergilli was offered by Stuart & Blank (1955) in Canada and by Gregson & La Touche (1961) in the United Kingdom where English & Dalton (1962) have reported a series of Aspergillus infections of post-operative aural cavities.

Mycotic abortion in cattle

Aspergilli together with a lengthy list of other common moulds, especially mucoraceous species, are also associated with abortion in cattle.[11] It was Theobald Smith (1920) in the United States who first recorded the isolation of a mould, identified as *Rhizopus rhizopodiformis* [*R. cohnii*] from the diseased foetal membranes and the amniotic fluid of a slaughtered pregnant cow. Five years later Gilman & Birch (1925) reported an unidentified species of *Mucor* associated with three cases of abortion in one herd and they were able to induce placental infection and abortion experimentally by intravenous injection of a suspension of the mould (Fig. 22). Bendixon & Plum (1929) monographed the disease on the basis of a study of 17 cases from which they isolated *Aspergillus fumigatus* (eight cases) or *Absidia ramosa* (two cases), or both (seven cases). Up to the nineteen-fifties little attention was paid to these findings but the work has now been confirmed and extended. More than forty different moulds have been shown to be implicated in mycotic abortion, 638 cases having been

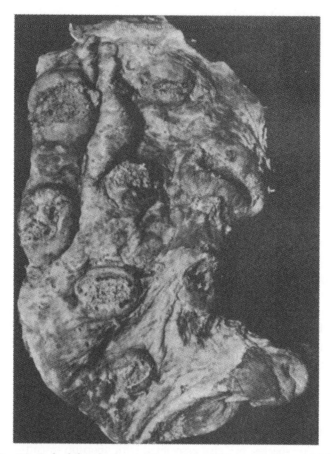

Fig. 22. End of the chorion in the non-gravid horn of a cow which aborted after experimental inoculation with a species of *Mucor*. The necrosis is quite well advanced and involved the inter-cotyledonous chorion. Note that the stems of all the cotyledons are necrotic, leaving typical crater-like depressions. (Gilman & Birch, 1925, Fig. 3).

diagnosed by Veterinary Investigation Officers and others in England and Wales during 1954–60, according to Austwick & Venn (1962).

Aspergillus nidulans has occasionally been found causing white-grained mycetoma and Dodge (1935) compiled more than thirty species of aspergilli considered to be pathogenic for man or animals but modern taxonomists would consign many of the names to synonymy and myco-pathologists would doubt the claim to pathogenic status of others. The position is similar for many other of the hyphomycetes which constitute what E. W. Mason called 'common mould', but on the other hand, as recounted in the next chapter, although there are few established pathogens there are many saprobic fungi of worldwide distribution in the environment able to infect man and higher animals under favourable circumstances.

While it is still a valid generalization that fungi are more important as pathogens of plants than of man and higher animals, statistics indicate that the incidence of fungal infection for the two groups of hosts is of the same order. For example, an examination of the index to Volume 4 of the *Review of Medical and Veterinary Mycology* covering 1961–3 showed 204 species of fungi recorded as pathogenic for man and 88 vertebrates; an average of 2.3 per host. The comparable figures for plant pathogenic fungi derived from the *Review of Applied Mycology* (in which the literature of plant pathology was surveyed) was 1288 fungi on 659 hosts; an incidence of approximately two species per host.[12] More recently, McGinnis (1980, Appendix A) reported the results, pointing in the same direction, of an interesting exercise in which he critically evaluated from the published data the pathogenic status of each of 278 species of fungi reported between the late 1940s to 1979 (when the evidence presented was much more reliable than for many earlier reports) as pathogenic for man. In making the assessments the four criteria to be met for pathogenic status to be accepted were: (1) an adequate clinical history suggesting a mycotic infection; (2) the fungus was seen in clinical specimens; (3) the morphology of the fungus in the clinical specimens was compatible with the reported aetiological agent; and (4) there was adequate evidence that the fungus was correctly identified. Of the 607 reports considered (representing 278 fungal taxa at 1–10 reports per taxon) 226 were rejected, the 381 accepted representing 174 fungi which is comparable to the number claimed as pathogenic for a staple crop plant.

5

Epidemiological problems

It is becoming platitudinous to recall that an infectious disease is not a static but a dynamic relationship involving the response of the host to the pathogen and the mirror image that of the pathogen to the host while both pathogen and host and their interaction are influenced by the external environment. Epidemiology, here taken in a broad sense to cover the totality of these relationships and not limited to the study of epidemics, is reviewed in this chapter by considering a series of interactions the analysis of some of which has been a major preoccupation during the last half-century.

1. Effects of the pathogen on the host

Knowledge of the effect of the pathogen on the host, which varies from minimal to fatal, has gradually accumulated over the centuries. For some two thousand years the only recorded effect of fungal infection of man was the *cutaneous* as typified by ringworm and candidosis of the skin and mucous membranes. It was not until the nineteenth century that more *superficial* infections were identified. In 1846 pityriasis versicolor, a mild noninflammatory infection of the stratum corneum, was first differentiated by Eichsted and described the following year by Sluyter in his doctoral thesis. Robin (1853) named the causal organism *Microsporum furfur* which is now classified in the genus *Malasezzia* along with the allied *M. ovale* found on the scalp in association with dandruff but now usually regarded as non-pathogenic. (In passing it is interesting to note that the latter was shown by Benham (1939) to have an obligate growth requirement for fatty acids.) Even more superficial are the two types of piedra, the name by which the black variety was known in Colombia where a clinical study of the infection was made in 1876 by Nicolau Ozorio and Pozada Arango who sent material to, among other European dermatologists, Desenne, Malcolm Morris, Juhel-Renay, and Behrend, all of whom published notes on the condition.[1] Black piedra was subsequently

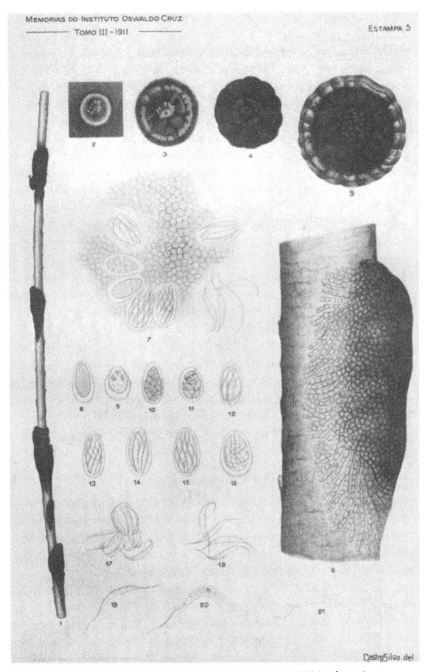

Fig. 23. Black piedra (*Piedraia hortae*). (Horta, 1911, plate v).

studied in Brazil by Horta (1911) and others, and the fungus responsible named *Trichosporon hortai* by Brumpt in 1913, and reclassified in a new genus as *Piedraia hortae* by Fonseca & Arêa Lêao (1928). In this disease, which occurs in tropical countries affecting both man and other primates such as chimpanzees (Kaplan, 1959*a*), the only signs are hard black nodules firmly attached to the shafts of scalp hair.[2] These nodules, up to one millimetre or so in diameter, are colonies of the pathogen within which its life cycle is completed by the production of ascospores (Fig. 23). The similar white piedra (*Trichosporon beigelii*), first recorded in Europe by Beigel (1865) on hair of a chignon, occurs in both tropical and temperate regions affecting man, the horse, and, in one instance noted by Kaplan (1959*b*), a monkey. The nodules are soft, pale in colour, and only arthrospores and blastospores are produced (Rabenhorst, 1867). These two series of infections are supplemented by a group of *subcutaneous* mycoses, including sporotrichosis, mycetomas, chromoblastomycosis, and rhinosporidiosis, which connect cutaneous infections with the climax provided by the major *systemic* mycoses histoplasmosis, blastomycosis, paracoccidioidomycosis, cryptococcosis, and coccidioidomycosis all of which are considered in greater detail later in this chapter.

Although fungal infection is frequently confined to the skin, hair, and nails, or has a cutaneous aspect, almost every organ of the body may suffer attack; the hands and the feet, the ear, nose, and eye; internally the lungs are most frequently involved but the lymphatics, brain, liver, kidneys and cebrospinal fluid do not escape. In cattle the udder may exhibit mastitis and infection of the placenta results in abortion while the air sacs of birds are commonly invaded.

Tissue response

The tissue response is equally varied. Erythema is characteristic of dermatophyte infections which may result in hyperkeratosis and keloid formations. In subcutaneous and systemic infections pyrogenic reactions are frequent as are granulomatous responses among many others which are tabulated by Rippon (1982:6). In microscopical preparations fungi may be differentiated by standard haematoxylin–eosin staining but this technique has been superseded by the periodic-acid–Schiff stain (based on the Feulgen reaction) introduced by Kligman & Mescon (1950) and the development of special stains for fungi such as the Gridley (1953) and Grocott (1955) staining procedures, the last being based on Gomori's methenamine–silver nitrate technique (Gomori, 1946). Gram staining is important for actinomycetes. *Actinomyces* and *Nocardia* are Gram-positive.

Immunological response

Fungi are antigenic and an important response of the infected host is the production of antibodies the reaction of which with their corresponding antigens may be detected by the various techniques developed by bacteriologists and virologists. These include complement fixation (a sensitive if rather complicated test), agglutination of particles of the antigen which may be fungal cells or collodion, latex, or bentonite particles on which antigen has been absorbed, or the formation of a precipitate on mixing solutions of antigen and antibody which may be observed directly or, as in the much used Ouchterlony technique (Fig. 24), by the formation of precipitation lines in agar gels. Recently the use of immunofluorescence, and the ELISA (enzyme-linked immunosorbent assay) test in particular, has become a popular method for detecting and quantifying antibodies. Much attention has been, and still is, paid to the serology of mycoses and much useful data has been obtained but for various reasons the serological approach to mycopathology has not attained the dominating importance of the technique in bacteriology and virology. One reason is that fungi are relatively weak antigens. Another that different pathogenic fungi have antigens in common so that there are cross-reactions between the antigens of one fungus with heterologous antisera. This has been used to assess phylogenetic relationships within the Fungi but, in general, serology remains unreliable for specific identification.

Perhaps the most useful serological contribution to the understanding of mycotic infection has been the exploitation of cellular bound, delayed type cutaneous hypersensitivity, a long-term skin sensitivity resulting from infection so that an antigenic preparation of the pathogen injected intradermally induces an area of induration (frequently associated with erythema) within 48 h indicating infection or previous infection of the subject tested. This phenomenon also underlies allergy to fungus spores (see Chapter 7).

Dermatophytoses. During the first decade of the present century the Swiss worker Bloch found that guinea pigs, after recovery from an experimental infection with either *Trichophyton quinckeanum* or *T. mentagrophytes*, were immune for as long as a year and a half to reinfection with the same fungus. He found that immunity, which was correlated with a hypersensitivity of the skin, could be induced only by cutaneous inoculation: subcutaneous or intraperitoneal injection of the living fungus or an extract of the fungus did not give rise to immunity or skin sensitivity.

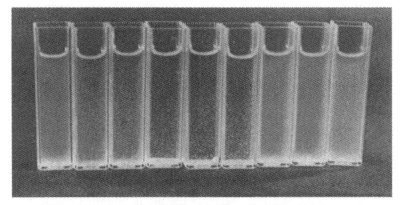

A Tube agglutination test for antibodies to *C. albicans*. The left-hand tube is a negative control, containing a suspension of killed *C. albicans* blastospores but no serum. In the remaining tubes, from left to right, suspensions of killed *C. albicans* were mixed with doubling dilutions of serum from a patient with systemic candidosis, beginning with a 1:10 dilution in the tube second from the left. Macroscopically visible agglutination of the *C. albicans* was achieved by serum dilutions up to 1:160. The agglutination titre of the patient's serum was therefore reported as 1:160.

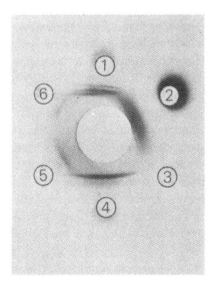

B Ouchterlony double diffusion test for precipitating antibodies to *Candida* antigens. Serum from a patient with systemic candidosis was placed in the centre, large well, cut in an agar gel. The surrounding small wells were filled with various soluble Candida extracts:

1. *C. albicans* culture filtrate, 2 mg/ml;
2. *C. albicans* 'cytoplasmic' antigen, 10 mg/ml;
3. saline solution (negative control);
4. *C. albicans* culture filtrate, 20 mg/ml;
5. *C. albicans* 'cytoplasmic' antigen, 1 mg/ml;
6. purified *C. albicans* mannan, 5 mg/ml. Note the presence of lines of identity and of nonidentity between the different antigens. The characteristically diffuse appearance of anti-mannan precipitin (seen most clearly in the reaction with well 5) has been referred to by some authorities as an 'H-type' appearance, by contrast with the sharp 'R-type' lines seen with protein antigens. The plate was stained with coomassie brilliant blue RL.

Fig. 24. Detection and quantification of antibodies by the Agglutination test (*A*); the Ouchterlony double diffusion test (*B*); Counter immunoelectrophoresis (*C*); and the Antigen-antibody crossed immunoelectrophoresis test (*D*). (Odds (1979): 213–14).

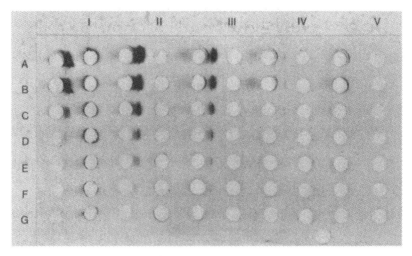

C Precipitating antibodies to *C. albicans* 'cytoplasmic' antigens detected by counter immunoelectrophoresis. Well rows A to G in alternate columns were filled with doubling dilutions of patient's serum (undiluted serum at top), while the well columns labelled I to V were each filled with 10-fold dilutions of *C. albicans* cytoplasmic antigen (10 mg of protein/ml in column I). The lines of precipitation, revealed by staining with coomassie brilliant blue HL, were formed after only 1½ hours of electrophoresis (anode at left). On a 'box titration' plate of this type, it is possible to assess the maximum number of precipitin lines formed by a patient's serum (there are at least eight lines adjacent to well pair AII), and the maximum precipitin titre (at least one precipitin line is still apparent in a dilution of 1:32 – well pairs FII and FIII). Counter immunoelectrophoresis therefore offers clear possibilities for both speed and quantitation in the Candida precipitin test.

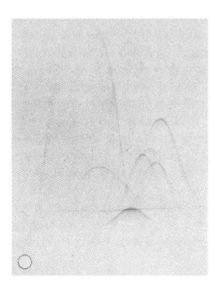

D 'Antigen–antibody crossed immunoelectrophoresis' in the detection of precipitating antibodies to Candida in this two-dimensional system. *C. albicans* 'cytoplasmic' antigen mixture was first electrophoresed across the plate from the well at bottom left. The plate was then turned through 90°, and now separated antigenic components were forced to migrate electrophoretically into a field of agarose containing serum from a patient with systemic candidosis. The precipitin peaks (revealed by staining the plate with coomassie brilliant blue RL) are the result of individual antigen–antibody reactions. The area of each peak is proportional to the relative concentrations of antigen and antibody. This system, although more tedious in technical performance, allows the resolution and identification of each individual anti-Candida precipitin in a patient's serum.

Further, Bloch sensitized himself by inoculation with *T. quinckeanum* and then grafted a piece of his skin and a piece of skin from a non-sensitized person over an ulcer on the leg of a third subject. Subsequent testing with a *Trichophyton* extract gave a positive reaction on the skin taken from Bloch but not on the skin of the control graft or on the skin of the patient (see Bloch, 1921, 1928).

Early attempts to demonstrate agglutinins, precipitins, and complement-fixing antibodies in ringworm infections were unsuccessful. This, as Conant *et al.* (1944) suggested, was in part a result of inadequate technique and recently improved methods of extraction and fractionation of dermatophyte antigens and the refinement of *in vitro* serological tests have shown that circulating antifungal antibodies are more prevalent during active dermatophyte infections than was generally believed (see Lepper, 1969).

It was Neisser and Plato in 1902 who first made an extract of a ringworm fungus, which they named *trichophytin* (of which the active principle is a galactomannan-peptide according to Barker *et al.*, 1963) and which on introduction into a patient suffering from ringworm caused a local erythematous response accompanied by a rise in temperature. Bloch found that the cutaneous response to trichophytin appeared a week or so after infection, an observation since confirmed by others who have shown that the skin sensitivity is sometimes retained for many years.

This skin sensitivity resulting from dermatophyte infection may result naturally in generalized signs in some infected subjects; a condition first noted by Jadssohn, in 1911, who described follicular eruptions in patients with kerion. These eruptions or *dermatophids*, which are sometimes distinguished as *trichophytids* and *microsporids* according to the genus of dermatophyte involved, occur on the body, the feet and legs, and, most frequently, the hands, and they disappear spontaneously on the elimination of the primary fungus infection. It is unusual for a fungus to be isolated from a dermatophytid which is thought to be an allergic response to the systemic spread of some metabolic product of the fungus, or perhaps fungus spores or elements, for there are a number of records of the isolation of ringworm fungi from the blood.

Peck (1950) offered evidence that sensitization to dermatophytes (some of which produce penicillin) is one of the factors determining sensitivity to penicillin, the injection of which sometimes gives rise to a reaction simulating that to trichophytin.

Candidiosis. Candida infections are also sometimes associated with allergic skin eruptions (*candidids*) which were first reported by Ravaut & Rabeau (1928–9) in France and Frost *et al.* (1929) in the United States and designated 'levurides' and 'moniliatids', respectively.

Coccidioidomycosis. In marked contrast to their employment for dermato-mycoses, skin sensitivity and other serological tests have given much help in deepening understanding of the incidence and treatment of systemic mycoses, especially coccidioidomycosis and histoplasmosis. Coccidioido-mycosis (*Coccidioides immitis*) was first recognized as a rare and frequently fatal generalized mycosis, originally described from South America and apparently endemic in southern California where from 1915 E. C. Dickson studied the condition and drew attention to the presence of healed pulmonary lesions, mimicking those of tuberculosis, which suggested that there was a milder form of the disease. Investigations in 1936 by Myrnie Gifford on a respiratory disease known in California as 'San Joaquin Valley fever' (and also as 'desert rheumatism' and 'the bumps' because of joint pains accompanied by erythema nodosum, particularly on anterior tibial areas, and erythema multiforme on the upper half of the body), showed it to be a benign form of coccidioidomycosis common in the region (see Dickson, 1937; Dickson & Gifford, 1938) which conferred immunity to subsequent infection. In 1927 Hirsch and Benson had demonstrated that skin hypersensitivity developed after infection by *C. immitis* and later a liquid asparagine-containing synthetic medium for the preparation of the antigen, which became available commercially as *coccidioidin*, was described by Charles E. Smith (1943) (Fig. 25) who, after joining the Dickson-Gifford team made the study of coccidioidomycosis in California his lifework.

Smith's studies were precipitated by observations during the 1939–45 war that coccidioidin sensitivity developed in troops stationed for training in desert regions of the United States and the finding that this was the result of suffering from primary coccidioidomycosis. At Florence, Arizona, a prisoner of war camp was closed because of the risk of infection to the nonimmune. Smith did more than anyone to establish the endemicity of coccidioidomycosis throughout the desert regions of California and the neighbouring states. He combed the deserts in an old Ford car, nicknamed 'the flying chlamydospore', and was fêted for his achievements at the second coccidioidomycosis conference of 1965 (Ajello, 1967).

The incidence of infection in endemic areas as gauged by the coccidioidin

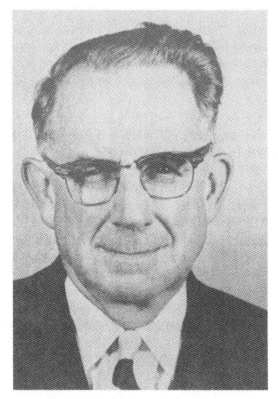

Fig. 25. Charles E. Smith (1904–67).

test is high. In South Arizona more than 97% of Indian children were found to give a positive reaction and throughout the region the number of reactors increased after dust storms and with the length of time resident in the area. Domesticated animals were also found to be susceptible. In cattle (for which Maddy et al., (1960) found the annual conversion rate to a positive skin reaction was almost identical to the human rate) the infection is usually benign and many cases were only recorded in slaughtered animals by meat inspectors (e.g. Prchal, 1948). In dogs Converse & Reed (1966) noted that most infections occurred during the cooler months, in contrast to the warm season pattern in man, and they suggested that this may be due to the dog's habit of digging burrows.

In addition to skin hypersensitivity, infection by C. immitis may result in the production of both precipitins and complement-fixing antibodies as was shown by C. E. Smith and his collaborators who in 1956 reported the results of 39 500 serological tests. Skin sensitivity usually begins to develop at two to 21 days after the appearance of symptoms, precipitins appear during the first to third weeks, and complement-fixing antibodies (when they occur) not until three months after the first symptoms. A high or rising titre of the last indicates a poor prognosis (Emmons et al., 1963).

Histoplasmosis, intracellular infection of the reticuloendothelial system by Histoplasma capsulatum, shows certain resemblances to coccidioidomycosis. Both diseases were first attributed to protozoa (see Chapter 1), both were considered to be rare diseases and usually fatal, and both within the past fifty years have been shown to be common non-contagious diseases, with a primary phase which is usually benign and confers immunity to reinfection which is rare for coccidioidomycosis (Winn, 1967) but more frequently reported for histoplasmosis (Schwarz & Baum, 1963; Powell et al., 1973). For histoplasmosis, like coccidioidomycosis, skin sensitivity testing made a major contribution to establishing the significance of the disease.

The first case of histoplasmosis was recognized post mortem in 1905 but it was not until 1934 that Katherine Dodd (at Vanderbildt University Nashville, Tennessee) diagnosed the first case (in an infant) ante mortem (to which DeMonbreun (1934) contributed the mycology and established the dimorphism of the pathogen) and by 1945 only 17 cases had been recorded world wide (see Parsons & Zarafonetis, 1945). A decade later it was estimated[3] conservatively that 25 to 30 million of the inhabitants of the Mississippi-Ohio River Valley had been infected by Histoplasma and that in eight states of the region a total of 800 deaths from histoplasmosis occurred annually. It had become apparent from radiological examinations that particularly in the Mississippi-Ohio valley there were many individuals who though tuberculin-negative showed small calcifications in the lungs. Tested with coccidioidin many reacted positively if a strong concentration of the antigen was used. No evidence of Coccidioides infection could be found and it was C. E. Smith who suggested that perhaps the positive reaction to coccidioidin was a cross-reaction with another fungus, possibly H. capsulatum. Histoplasmin testing by Palmer (1945), Christie & Peterson (1945), and others (see Iams (1950) who summarized 27 780 recorded tests) quickly established the correctness of this suggestion and a correlation between the presence of lung calcifications in tuberculin-negative individuals. In addition, a positive response to histoplasmin by those lacking pulmonary calcifications indicated that, like coccidioidomycosis, histoplasmosis had a mild form. These findings – which were amply confirmed – aroused much interest and Norman Conant arranged a

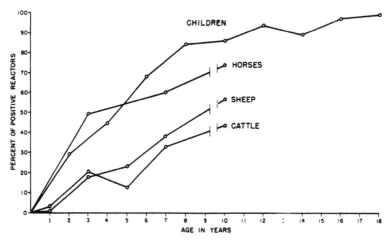

Fig. 26. Incidence of histoplasmosis in children and farm animals in relation to age. (Furcolow, 1958).

seminar on histoplasmosis at the National Institutes of Health in September 1948 and M. L. Furcolow, who had set up a centre in Kansas City for the study of histoplasmosis in 1945, organized national conferences in 1952 and 1962.[4] Summaries of the extensive literature were later produced in book form and a succession of review articles (see introduction to Bibliography).

Domesticated animals are exposed to the same hazard of contracting histoplasmosis as man and Menges (1954) recorded sensitivity rates of 5% for cattle, 73% for horses, 33% for sheep, 1% for pigs, and 1% for chickens in Kansas, Missouri, and Iowa. He also recorded a 14% incidence in a random sample of 102 dogs from Kansas and Missouri while Furcolow & Ruhe (1949) found a close similarity between the positive reaction rates of children and cattle of successive age groups of one to seven years (see Fig. 26).

As for coccidioidomycosis, precipitins and complement-fixing antibodies also result but because of cross-reactions with the antigens of *Blastomyces dermatitidis* (blastomycosis) serological tests, though useful, have to be interpreted with caution (see Campbell, 1960); and even greater caution is needed for candidosis and aspergillosis.

2. Effects of the host on the pathogen

Most fungal pathogens of man and higher animals are mycelial (fila-mentous) in the saprobic state while a few are yeasts (single cells reproducing by budding). It is very rare for the pathogenic state to duplicate the saprobic but *Aspergillus fumigatus*, for which only a conidial (anamorphic) state is known, may be found growing in the air sacs of birds (Owen, 1832) or the respiratory passages of mammals (Rewell & Ainsworth, 1947) as a greenish sporulating felt indistinguishable from an *in vitro* culture. Further, *A. niger* and, less frequently, *A. fumigatus*, sometimes form masses of fungal hyphae and cell debris (known as 'fungus balls' or *aspergillomas*). 1–5 cm in diameter, in ectatic bronchi or cavities resulting from other diseases (e.g. old tuberculosis cavities), and, but rarely, other sites such as the bladder. Such aspergillomas, first differentiated by Dévé (1938), may also exhibit typical sporulation on their exposed surfaces.

Usually the pathogenic phase is characterized by a more restricted growth than the saprobic. *Cryptococcus neoformans* (cryptococcosis) in which the single vegetative cells *in vitro*, if less-frequently capsulated, correspond to the capsulated cells of the pathogenic phase, whether in tissue or cerebrospinal fluid, is only known to produce the teleomorphic basidiomycetous state in culture. Dermatophytes are mycelial anamorphic fungi with or without associated teleomorphic states but pathogenic growth in skin is usually restricted to sterile mycelium and sporulation on or in hairs limited to microconidia although, as first recorded by Plaut (1902) and independently demonstrated by Davidson and Gregory in Canada in 1933, macroconidia and other characteristic morphological structures develop on detached hairs held under conditions of high humidity.

As noted in Chapter 2, Gruby's interpretation of the relationship of the dermatophyte to the hair was an error. He believed that the fungus grew upwards from the bulb into the hair. It was fifty years later that H. G. Adamson, a London dermatologist (Fig. 27), showed in detail that the dermatophyte is confined to the keratinized portion of the hair and that the direction of growth is downwards towards the bulb. The downward-growing hyphae do not penetrate the bulb but terminate above it in a fringe of hyphal endings, known as 'Adamson's fringe' (Fig. 28), the downward growth of which keeps pace with the elongation and keratiniza-tion of the hair shaft. That dermatophytes utilize keratinized tissue can readily be shown by offering horn as the sole nutrient. Observations on

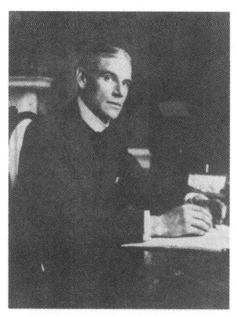

Fig. 27. H. G. Adamson (1865–1955). (Wellcome Institute Library, London).

the invasion of hairs at right angles to their length by special 'penetrating organs' which cause round-bottomed pits in the hair as first described by Davidson & Gregory (1934) and in greater detail by Vanbreuseghem (1949) and others (especially English (1963, 1968) who reviews the topic) strongly suggest enzyme involvement although attempts to isolate a keratolytic enzyme have been unsuccessful. An important post-war investigation on the pathogenicity of ringworm fungi was that by Albert M. Kligman (University of Pennsylvania School of Medicine) on tinea capitis caused by *Microsporum audouinii* and *M. canis* in which studies similar to those of Adamson and Sabouraud were made by the experimental inoculation of children, the progress of infection being studied by biopsy material subjected to modern histological techniques (Kligman, 1952, 1955). He distinguished four phases of experimental tinea capitis which are summarized in Table 2.

Kligman also investigated ringworm infection in the mouse, rat, and hamster in which the hair growth is cyclic and found that susceptibility to infection coincided with the second half of the growth period (Kligman, 1956).

British Journal of Dermatology.] [Vol. VII., No. 7.

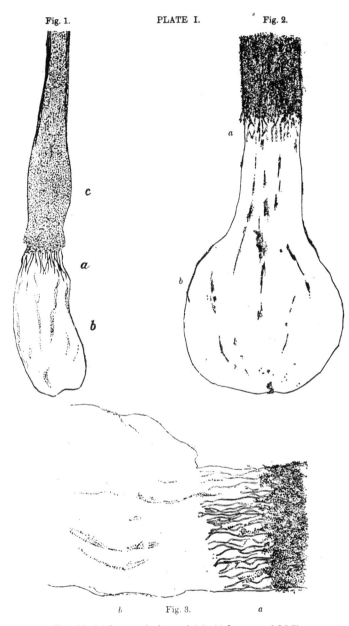

Fig. 1. PLATE I. Fig. 2.

Fig. 3.

Fig. 28. 'Adamson's fringe' (a). (Adamson, 1895).

Table 2. *The four phases of tinea capitis* (Kligman, 1955)

	Clinical Observations	Microscopic Observations
Incubation period (2 to 4 days)	No gross evidence of disease	Hyphae in stratum corneum and follicular orifice: hyphae grow downward into the follicle on the hair's surface; the intrafollicular hyphae break up into chains of cells (primary spore formation)
Period of spread (4 days to 4 mo.)	Individual lesions enlarge radially and new lesions continue to appear; newly infected hairs when plucked show a band of fluorescence at the base; fluorescence reaches scalp surface about 12th day; at about 3 wk. hairs break off a few millimetres above scalp surface	Fungus proliferates in the stratum corneum and invades new follicles in its radial path of growth; intrafollicular hyphae penetrate hair on 6th to 7th day; intrapilary hyphae descend to exact upper limit of keratogenous zone and here form Adamson's fringe (about 12th day); external branches of the intrapilary hyphae segment into short chains of ectothrix spores
Refractory period (4 mo. to several yr.)	No new lesions develop; clinical appearance constant throughout this period; host and parasite at equilibrium	Hyphae no longer present in stratum corneum; anatomical relationship of fungus to hair remains constant; intrapilary hyphae never penetrate into keratogenous zone or bulb of hair; large quantities of ectothrix spores formed
Period of involution	Individual hairs show diminished fluorescence; hairs become longer and break less readily	Formation of ectothrix spores gradually ceases; quantity of intrapilary hyphae progressively reduced

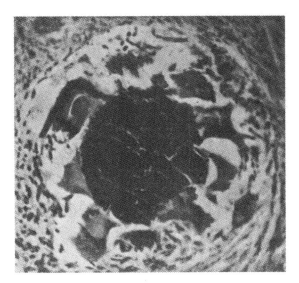

Fig. 29. Black grain of *Madurella mycetomatis* (Laveran) Brumpt in tissue. × 165. (Brumpt, 1906, plate xx, fig. 2).

Granules

Except in terminal conditions, it is unusual for a mycelial pathogen to spread freely through infected tissue. Aspergillus infection of the lung, udder, or other tissue, for example, is usually limited by the reaction of the host cells as shown by the swollen hyphal tips of the pathogen and its restriction to a more or less spherical growth resembling a colony of a shaken culture. Similar effects are shown by other pathogenic fungi, and also actinomycetes. When there is abscess formation, the embedded colonies of the pathogen may be discharged in the pus as small particles ('grains' or 'granules') which are frequently of diagnostic value (Fig. 29).

The two best known diseases characterized by grains are mycetoma (monographed by Mahgoub & Murray, 1973) and actinomycosis (monographed by Cope, 1938; Bronner & Bronner, 1969). The former was known in ancient India (as noted in Chapter 1) and in recent times was first recognized by British surgeons of the Indian Medical Service. Gill, of Madura, Madras, in his Dispensary Report of 1842 drew attention to a disease of the foot characterized by marked deformity, large fungoid excrescences, and the discharge of a thick ichorous fluid. The same disease was reported six years later by J. Colebrook, also of Madura, who noted that the disease was commonly known in parts of southern India as 'Madura foot'. Shortly afterwards, Henry Vandyke Carter, of Bombay,

made a special investigation of the condition (which he designated
mycetoma) and later presented the results in a comprehensive and hand-
some monograph (Carter, 1874). The foot is the usual site of infection
although the hand or other part is sometimes involved. A localized lesion
spreads to cause tumefaction and deformity with multiple abscesses which
are drained by fistulae (see Frontispiece). The pus contains minute
granules which sometimes provide a clue to the identity of the pathogen
involved for although mycetoma is a very characteristic clinical entity it
is not, as Carter was the first to recognize, an aetiological entity, some forty
organisms classified in a dozen genera have been claimed as causally
related to the condition. Carter submitted specimens to the Rev. Miles
Joseph Berkeley, the leading English mycologist to the time, who obtained
from the material a new but now unidentifiable saprobic mould which in
1863 he named *Chionyphe carteri*. The identity of the causal agents was
not elucidated until the turn of the century. Aetiologically there are two
main series of mycetomas, one caused by fungi, the other by aerobic
actinomycetes such as *Actinomadura madurae* first reported by Vincent
(1894) as *Streptothrix madurae*. Pinoy (1913) separated mycetomas caused
by actinomycetes as 'actinomycoses' from 'true mycetomas' caused by
fungi such as species of *Madurella* described by Brumpt (1905, 1906) in
his important monograph. Later Chalmers & Archibald (1916, 1918) at
the Wellcome Tropical Research Laboratories in the Sudan where interest
in mycetoma has persisted (see Abbott, 1956), in a comprehensive review
of the subject introduced 'maduromycosis' for Pinoy's second category.
Today *actinomycosis* is reserved for conditions caused by anaerobic (microaerophilic) actinomycetes and the two series of mycetomas differentiated
by the terms *eumycetoma* and *actinomycetoma*.

Carter (1874) distinguished 'melanoid' and 'ochroid' variations of
mycetoma according to the colour of the granules. Black-grained
mycetoma caused by *Madurella mycetomatis* may be considered the classic
variety but black grains are also produced by species of *Penicillium* and
Phialophora. Species of *Aspergillus, Cephalosporium, Indiella*, and *Psudal-
lescheria* give white grains while those of actinomycetes (*Actinomadura,
Streptomyces, Nocardia*) vary from white through yellow and orange to red.
Microscopic examination readily distinguishes fungal from actinomycotic
granules.

The cervicofacial form of classical actinomycosis (caused by species of
Actinomyces, a genus now reserved for microaerophilic species) has been
well documented for the past century as 'lumpy jaw' of cattle and man;
as have the less-frequent infections at other sites in man, cattle and a

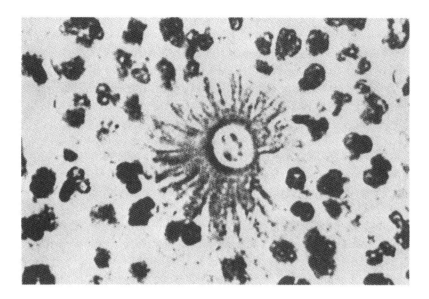

Fig. 30. Asteroid body of *Sporothrix schenckii* lying among pus cells.
(*Sporotrichosis infection...*, 1947, fig. 5).

range of domestic animals. All such infections are characterized by the
presence in the associated pus of yellowish grains or 'sulphur granules'.
It was Wolff & Israel (1891) who first obtained cultures of the causal
anaerobe which modern studies (Lord, 1910, and extended by Emmons,
1938) have shown to be present in the normal mouth and the tonsillar
crypts. It is from such sources that infection originates; it is not carried
to the mouth by straws (which are frequently contaminated by aerobic
actinomycetes) as was formerly supposed but a lesion caused by chewing
straw could provide an entry for the pathogen.

Asteroids

Mention may appropriately be made of structures bearing a certain
resemblance to granules which are occasionally found in invaded tissues
and variously known as 'asteroids' or 'asteroid bodies' (Fig. 30). Asteroid
bodies were first observed by Splendore (1908) in Brazil in human
sporotrichotic material. They have been reported by many authors since
and today their presence is generally accepted as presumptive evidence for
a diagnosis of sporotrichosis. From a light- and electron-microscopic study
Lurie & Still (1969) concluded that the apparent capsule seen surrounding
a yeast-like cell of *Sporothrix schenckii* in some fixed preparations is an

artifact and that the asteroid body is formed by the precipitation of an antigen–antibody complex which is deposited on the surface of the cell, increases in amount, and becomes star-shaped. Austwick (1962) described asteroids 50–80 μm in diameter associated with swollen hyphae of *Aspergillus fumigatus* in lung lesions of dairy cows, the eosinophilic asteroid sheath being of crystalline structure.

Dimorphism[5]

The effect of the host on the pathogen that has generated most interest is dimorphism which, in this connection, may be defined as the occurrence of a fungus having a mycelial phase as yeast-like (or non-mycelial) in the host. This phenomenon is particularly associated with a group of systemic mycoses of man and animals first described from the Americas. In coccidioidomycosis (*Coccidioides immitis*), described from Argentina in 1892, and histoplasmosis (*Histoplasma capsulatum*), described from the Panama Canal Zone in 1905–6, the pathogens were, as noted in Chapter 1, at first mistaken for protozoa. Blastomycosis (widely referred to as North American blastomycosis (*Blastomyces dermatitidis*) (Fig. 52) was first recorded as 'blastomycetic dermatitis' by Gilchrist (1896) in the United States and for some years, as 'Gilchrist's disease', confused with coccidioidomycosis (see Benham, 1934), cryptococcosis ('torulosis') (*Cryptococcus neoformans*) (see Conant, 1939) and also with paracoccidioidomycosis (South American blastomycosis) (*Paracoccidioides brasiliensis*) described by Lutz (1908) from Brazil as 'pseudococcidioides granuloma'. Another member of this group is sporotrichosis (*Sporothrix schenckii*), a mycosis of worldwide distribution first described in man, by Schenck (1898) in the United States, rats (*Mus decumanus*) in Brazil (Lutz & Splendore, 1907), and horses, in Madagascar by Carougeau (1909) as *Sporotrichum equi* (a synonym of *Sporothrix schenckii* fide Hyde & Davis, 1910).

There has been much investigation of the conditions which control the mycelial-yeast (yeast–mycelial) (M$\rightleftharpoons$Y) transformation. Romano[6] in his general review distinguished three categories of dimorphism: temperature dependent, temperature and nutrition dependent, and nutrition dependent. The simplest example of dimorphism and the first to be noted, by Hamberger as long ago as 1907, is that of *B. dermatitidis* (blastomycosis) which is controlled by temperature alone. When cultured *in vitro* at 37 °C the growth is yeast-like, at 25 °C mycelial (Levine & Ordal, 1946); (in his thesis of 1931 (University of Buenos Aires)) and Negroni and Salvin (1949) showed that *P. brasiliensis* (paracoccidioidomycosis) behaves in a similar manner. These two transformations occur on minimal medium, usually the medium has to be enriched and there is frequently a requirement for increased carbon dioxide. The yeast phase of *S. schenckii* (sporotrichosis) was obtained by Drouhet & Mariat (1952) by incubation at 37 °C on an inorganic nitrogen-containing medium under 5% carbon dioxide and Bullen (1949) found that the mycelial–yeast transformation of *Histoplasma farciminosum* (epizootic lymphangitis of horses) occurred best at 37 °C on blood agar of pH 7.4 in an atmosphere containing 15–20% carbon dioxide. The Y⇌M conversion of *H. capsulatum* (histoplasmosis) is easily effected by reducing the temperature from 37 °C to 25 °C but the M→Y transformation *in vitro* has proved difficult. Conant (1941) effected this transformation on blood agar in tubes sealed with paraffin wax, while Campbell (1947) used a cysteine-blood medium; Pine & Peacock (1958) claimed that the mycelial phase is inhibited by citrate, and that calcium and magnesium reverse the effects of citric acid, magnesium stimulating and calcium inhibiting M→Y. More recently Hempel & Goodman (1975) obtained the yeast phases of *H. capsulatum*, *B. dermatitidis*, and *S. schenckii* in tissue culture of guinea pig peritoneal macrophage.

Two other examples of dimorphism in pathogenic fungi, *Candida albicans* (candidosis) and *Coccidioides immitis* (coccidioidomycosis), are of particular interest. In culture a blastospore of *C. albicans* may multiply by budding to give a yeast growth. Sometime the bud may elongate, produce from its tip a second elongated bud which repeats the process and as this succession of cells remain attached to one another a hypha-like structure (*pseudohypha*) results. Alternatively, the blastospore may germinate to produce a system of branching septate hyphae. In hyphae blastospores or hyphal branches develop behind septa and in pseudohyphae blastospores or elongated buds are similarly produced behind the constrictions which occur at the septal junctions. Another *in vitro* feature of *C. albicans* which is of diagnostic value is the production of thick-walled resting spores (chlamydospores). *In vivo* and *in vitro* one or other form may predominate and it was Audry (1887) in France who first proved that only one fungus was involved and that its manifestation depended on the growth medium. Since then much investigation, concisely reviewed by Odds (1979: 31–41), has been devoted to determining the conditions controlling the morphogenesis of *C. albicans* and the relationship of the different morphological forms to pathogenicity. At one time the view was widely held that it was to the ability to make mycelial growth that *C. albicans* owed its success as a pathogen but Odds concludes:

Recent work on *C. albicans* dimorphism *in vitro* suggests that hyphal formation is a gratuitous transitory response of the organism during growth under environmental condition of high temperature and neutral pH. Hyphal production *in vivo* is therefore probably similarly gratuitous and is an indication of active growth, but not necessarily of tissue invasion by the fungus. The appearance of hyphae in clinical material cannot therefore be regarded as absolute diagnostic evidence for candidosis...(Odds, 1979:40).

Coccidioides immitis, which is usually categorized as dimorphic, does not exhibit a mycelium–yeast transformation. In *in vitro* culture *C. immitis* develops as a mycelium bearing terminal chains of barrel-shaped arthro-conidia which readily separate and become airborne. On inhalation into the lungs of a susceptible host each arthroconidium increases in size to form a large spherical cell or 'spherule' (sporangium) the contents of which divide into numerous uninucleate sporangiospores which after rupture of the spherule wall spread into surrounding tissue and repeat the process. The usual response of the host is mild or subclinical but the condition may become acute and disseminated with a fatal result. An occasional spherule is found *in vitro* cultures where they may be consistently obtained on various media, especially variants of that devised by Converse (1955), and several authors, including Roberts, Counts & Creselius (1970), have advocated this as a method for confirming the identity of *C. immitis*.

While investigating the relationship of *C. immitis* to rodents Emmons found the lungs of these animals to be frequently infected by another interesting fungus which he and Ashburn (1942) considered to be an undescribed phycomycete which they assigned to the genus *Haplo-sporangium*. Ciferri and Montemartini disagreed with this disposition and in 1959 erected the new hyphomycete genus *Emmonsia* to which they transferred Emmons and Ashburn's species as *E. parva*. Subsequently a second species, *E. crescens*, was recognized but this is now awarded varietal status by some while others consider *Emmonsia* and *Chrysosporium* to be congeneric. Emmonsia infection is recognized by large vacuolated cells 20–40 µm (*E. parva*) or 200–700 µm (*E. crescens*) in diameter which recall *C. immitis* spherules. In culture Emmonsia is mycelial and bears smooth conidia of up to 3.5 or 4.5 µm diameter for the two variants. On being inhaled and lodging in the endobronchial alveolar spaces of the lung each spore (*adiaspore*, adiaconidium; hence the disease name *adiaspiro-mycosis*) merely increases in size and initiates a return to the mycelial state on death and decomposition of the host. The host response to infection is minimal to granulomatous. The disease was found to be widespread and to occur in many kinds of animals including mice, rats, moles, rabbits, skunks, weasels, mink, armadillos, wallabies, and opposums; and Jellison (who monographed adiaspiromycosis in 1969) while examining specimens in a Stockholm museum found *E. crescens* in the preserved lungs of

Microtus agrestis trapped in 1845. The first modern record in rodents, from Transcaucasian USSR, is probably that by Kirschenblatt (1939).

Dimorphism is not restricted to pathogenic fungi and it is probable that many mycelial fungi have a potential for growth in a yeast form. For example, Bartnicki-Garcia and Nickerson in 1962[7] made a comprehensive study of the growth of saprobic species of *Mucor* as yeasts, a phenomenon dependent on the absence of oxygen and the presence of carbon dioxide. Earlier Nickerson & Mankowski (1953) found that filamentation of *Candida albicans*, favoured by a polysaccharide medium, was reversed by the addition of cysteine which they interpreted as supplying sulphydryl ($-SH$) groups necessary for optimum growth and cell division. The interpretation of dimorphism is not clear. It may well be a general response to unfavourable conditions. Some normally plant-parasitic fungi, such as Smuts (Ustilaginales), which are mycelial in the parasitic phase are yeast-like in artificial culture and as most of the systemic mycoses are exogenous a yeast form may be an important factor in allowing normally saprobic fungi to establish themselves in warm-blooded animals.

3. The pathogen and the environment

Although most fungi pathogenic for man and animals will grow saprobically and so are not, or not wholly, dependent on a host for survival there are few early records of such fungi found as saprobes in nature. Sanfelice in 1895 first described *Cryptococcus neoformans* (as *Saccharomyces neoformans*) from fruit juices in Italy, de Beurmann & Gougerot (1908) in France isolated *Sporothrix schenckii* (as *Sporotrichum beurmanni*) from beech bark and other plant material, and in 1932 Benham and Kesten showed *S. schenckii* to be pathogenic for carnations. Plant material contaminated by *S. schenckii* is thought to be the source of human and animal infections. Gastineau *et al.* (1941) recorded the isolation of *S. schenckii* from sphagnum moss associated with a small epidemic of sporotrichosis among florists while in gold mines in South Africa an epidemic of sporotrichosis – the largest ever recorded; see Chapter 6 – originated from infected mine timbers. In 1937, in England, Muende and Webb recorded *Trichophyton mentagrophytes* on cow dung and in the same year Conant in the United States identified *Phialophora verrucosa* (a cause of chromomycosis) with a fungus isolated from wood pulp but it was not until the recognition of the association of outbreaks of coccidioidomycosis with dust storms that attention was paid to the soil as a reservoir of fungi responsible for mycoses.

Soil

Stewart & Meyer (1932) were the first to isolate *Coccidioides immitis* from soil; from a ranch at Delano, California, on which there were four cases of coccidioidal granuloma (progressive coccidioidomycosis). Davis *et al.* (1942) isolated the same fungus from soil associated with a rattlesnake burrow (in the Panoche Valley, California) dug out by a party of students who subsequently developed primary coccidioidomycosis and Emmons (1942) isolated *C. immitis* from four random samples of desert soil collected near San Carlos, Arizona. There have been many more such reports which have helped to establish that the North American distribution of endemic coccidioidomycosis is coincident with the Lower Sanorian Life Zone of the United States and Mexico, a region of low rainfall, high summer temperature, and characteristic flora. Similar areas where coccidioidomycosis is endemic are to be found in Argentina, Paraguay, and Venezuela.

Other first records of pathogenic fungi from soil include *Histoplasma capsulatum* (Emmons, 1949), *Sporothrix schenckii* (Emmons, 1950), *Cryptococcus neoformans* (Emmons, 1951), *Nocardia asteroides* (Gordon & Hagan, 1936), *Pseudallescheria boydii* (Emmons, 1950; Ajello & Zeidberg, 1951), and *Blastomyces dermatitidis* (Denton *et al.*, 1961), all in North America, and *Candida albicans* from two samples of soil (one urban, the other from a stackyard) in New Zealand (di Menna, 1955).

Baiting soil or other substrata for the differential isolation of fungi, including keratinophilic fungi, had long been practised[8] but the introduction by Vanbreuseghem (1952) of baiting soil with hair for the specific purpose of isolating dermatophytes revealed the world wide occurrence of dermatophyte-like fungi which had hitherto escaped the notice of the many investigators of the microfungi of the soil and a large literature, much of it repetitive, quickly developed.

The series of geophilic dermatophytes (reviewed by Ajello, 1974), which supplement the anthropophilic and zoophilic series (see below) not found in soil, include species of both *Microsporum* and *Trichophyton*. Among these are *M. gypseum* (a well established pathogen of man and animals), *M. cookei* (widely distributed, frequently isolated from animal fur, occasionally as a pathogen), and *M. nanum* (the most common cause of ringworm in pigs). Prominent among the *Trichophyton* species are *T. terrestre* and *T. ajelloi* which are both cosmopolitan, frequently isolated from animal fur, and of low pathogenicity in contrast to the highly pathogenic tropical *T. simii* which has a wide host range.

Some pathogenic fungi found in soil have been shown to have associations with the droppings of animals; for example, *Histoplasma capsulatum* with old chicken manure (Zeidberg *et al.*, 1952) and with the droppings of bats (Emmons, 1958) and starlings (*Sturnus vulgaris*) (Ajello, 1964), and *Cryptococcus neoformans* with dry pigeon excreta (Emmons, 1955). Only for bats is it believed that infected animals contribute to the contamination of the excreta. Human epidemics have usually first drawn attention to the contaminated material.

The associations of histoplasmosis with bats and starlings attracted much interest. In 1948, Washburn, Tuohy and Davis described a pulmonary disorder they called 'cave sickness' in persons who had visited certain bat-infested caves and from soil from the mouth of one cave, an isolation of *H. capsulatum* was made. This epidemic was accepted by Grayston & Furcolow (1953) as one of histoplasmosis and subsequently confirmed outbreaks of histoplasmosis among speleologists have been reported from Venezuela and South Africa (Transvaal). In Peru, histoplasmosis, known locally as 'fiebre de Tingo Maria', was associated with a cave inhabited by nocturnal, fruit-eating 'oil birds' (*Steatornis caripensis*). The presence of Histoplasma in the cave soil was attributed to its enrichment by their droppings but the cave was also inhabited by bats. These cases are briefly reviewed by Emmons (1958) in a detailed report of a family outbreak of histoplasmosis in Maryland traced to bat guano produced by a colony of bats (*Eptesicus fuscus*) inhabiting the attic of the farmhouse.

An outbreak of pneumonia, attributed to *H. capsulatum*, among military personnel at Camp Gruber, Oklahoma, in the spring of 1944 was reported by Feller *et al.* (1956). The source of the outbreak was traced to an abandoned storm cellar; 31 of 42 persons visiting the cellar were known to have contracted the disease (most of the 27 hospitalized being severely affected) and four of the others had suggestive symptoms. The diagnosis of histoplasmosis was confirmed by serological testing of those affected and the isolation of *H. capsulatum* from cellar soil both directly and by animal inoculation.

It is the habit of starlings to assemble at night in very large numbers at roosting sites in trees and on buildings under which guano accumulates. Starlings were intentionally introduced into Central Park, New York, in 1890 and 1891. Within a few years they established themselves in the New York area from which they spread south and west to become a major nuisance and the population of starlings is now high in the states from Ohio to Missouri and south to Tennessee where histoplasmosis is endemic.

Dodge *et al.* (1965) reported an epidemic of histoplasmosis in school children associated with a starling roost which overhung the school playground. Many similar records followed. Negroni (1965) suggested that the lack of starlings was correlated with the lower incidence of histoplasmosis in Argentina but in Great Britain where the starling population is high the incidence of histoplasmosis is even lower. The histoplasma-containing guano, whether of starlings or chickens, is usually old and the presence of feathers may be of significance. Campbell, Hill & Falgout (1962) isolated *H. capsulatum* from a chicken-feather pillow associated with histoplasmosis in an infant and subsequently Campbell and others studied the growth of *H. capsulatum* on feathers.[9] It is interesting to note that C. D. Smith & Furcolow (1964) demonstrated growth-stimulating substances for *H. capsulatum* and *Blastomyces dermatitidis* in infusions of starling manure.

Water

Of the many and diverse fungi found in fresh water and the sea, the study of which is a currently popular mycological specialization, few have been noted as pathogenic for man or other vertebrates. The most notorious mycosis of fish is salmon disease associated with species of *Saprolegnia* and another mycosis of salmon and trout (and also wholly marine fish such as herrings) caused by *Ichthyophonus hoferi*, a fungus of uncertain affinity, has a wide distribution. Recently the isolation of *Loboa loboi* (the pathogen responsible for lobomycosis in man) from dolphins which spend part of their time in estuarine waters off the coast of Surinam (where lobomycosis is endemic) by De Vries & Laarman (1973) and the Florida coast of the United States (where it is not) by Migaki *et al.* (1971) and Caldwell *et al.* (1975) has attracted attention but the significance of these observations is unknown.

Saprolegnia infection of a roach in England was first described in 1748 (see Fig. 2) but saprolegniosis first attracted general notice in the United Kingdom as a result of a serious outbreak of salmon disease in the rivers Conway and Tweed in 1877. Worthington Smith (1878) writing in the *Gardeners' Chronicle* attributed the disease to *Saprolegnia ferax* while T. H. Huxley (1882), in an excursion into mycology as one of Her Majesty's Inspectors of Fisheries, identified the pathogen as *S. monoica*. In 1903 J. Hume Patterson, Assistant Bacteriologist to the Corporation of Glasgow, published the results of his experimental investigation into the cause of salmon disease from which he concluded that *S. ferax* was a secondary infection following attack by the bacterium '*Bacillus salmonis pestis*' which he considered to be the primary cause of the disease. Salmon disease was not epidemic at the time of this study and Patterson reports that he had great difficulty in obtaining material which could well have been of furunculosis, a widespread bacterial disease of salmon and trout caused by *Aeromonas salmonicida*, and the Saprolegnia indeed a secondary infection. Since then there has been a continuous series of records associating species of Saprolegnia with disease in various freshwater fish, in some cases with reports of confirmatory experimental infections. C. W. Coker differentiated the Saprolegnia associated with fish and fish eggs as *S. parasitica* for which Kanouse (1932) gave an emended description resulting from her experimental study in which she obtained evidence of pathogenicity for fish eggs while Tiffney (1939) in an investigation of the host range of *S. parasitica* summarized earlier reports. It appears that while some forms of the *parasitica–diclina* complex are pathogenic, others are not, and that the former exhibit specialization for different species of fish (Willoughby, 1978).

A mycosis of man and domesticated animals in which waterborne infection possibly plays a part is rhinosporidiosis caused by *Rhinosporidium seeberi*, another organism of uncertain provenance but possibly related to *Ichthyophonus hoferi*. The disease is characterized by the production of large polyps from mucocutaneous tissue, particularly of the nose, and these growths each contain many spherules which may finally attain a diameter of up to 350 μm and contain up to 20000 spores which are the infective agents. Rhinosporidiosis was first reported from Argentina by Posadas and independently by O'Kinealy (1903) from India (Madras) where the disease is of common occurrence. First thought to be caused by a protozoan but Ashworth (1923), who gave a detailed account of the life history (Fig. 31) based on the investigation of an infection in an Indian student at the University of Edinburgh, tentatively suggested a chytrid relationship and proposed the new genus *Rhinosporidium. R. seeberi* has never been cultured or recorded from nature. Not infrequently a series of infected individuals have been reported as using the same well or water tank and Mandlick (1937) recorded 20% infection among a group of men cleaning a river bed. Men are more usually infected than women; bullocks more frequently than cows. Rao (1938) in Madras noted that affected bullocks were four to nine years old. It is at about three and a half years of age that bullocks have the nasal septum punctured for the nose string and are set to the plough. Infection was commonly recorded on the margin

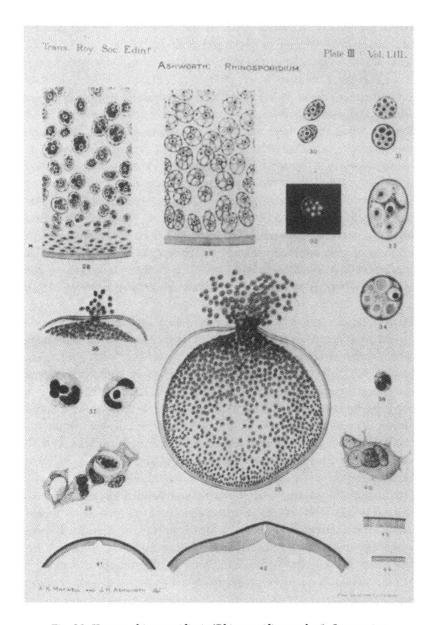

Fig. 31. Human rhinosporidiosis (*Rhinosporidium seeberi*). Sporangium and sporangiospores. (Ashworth, 1923, plate iii).

of the string hole. Cows are rarely used for ploughing. This suggests the possibility that bullocks and men contract the infection from a common source, possibly soil dust.

Animal hosts

The first records of mycotic disease in animals were those of saprolegniosis in fish and aspergillosis in birds as noted in Chapter 1. In general, the relationship of pathogenic fungi to their hosts is that some are adapted to parasitize man and are rarely, or less frequently, recorded from animals; others are adapted to parasitize animals and are rarely, or less frequently, recorded from man, while both man and animals are exposed to the hazard of infection by what are currently widely known as 'opportunitistic' fungi living saprobically in the environment. All three categories may be illustrated by the dermatophytes. *Epidermophyton floccosum* has only been recorded from human skin. *Microsporum audouinii*, the classical cause of head ringworm in children in western Europe and North America, has only rarely been recorded from animals. Although human infections by such zoophilic dermatophytes as the common cat and dog ringworm fungus, *M. canis*, and the cattle ringworm fungus, *Trichophyton verrucosum*, are of common occurrence such infections, if more inflammatory than those of typically anthropomorphilic dermatophytes, are usually limited and do not initiate large-scale epidemics. The geophilic *M. gypseum*, which has been found in soil from all parts of the world has also been reported sporadically from man and a diversity of animals but does not induce epidemic spread, may be cited as an example of the third group.

Farm and domestic animals, especially cattle, cats and dogs, when infected by dermatophytes provide reservoirs of infection for human ringworm and the question as to whether there were also reservoirs of infection among wild animals has attracted attention. In New Zealand Marples (1956) suggested that feral cats were a major factor in initiating outbreaks of *Microsporum canis* infection in man (and La Touche (see Chapter 6) attributed a similar role to domestic cats in an urban environment). Emmons (1942) at first thought that he had discovered an animal reservoir for coccidioidomycosis in Arizona when he found that desert rodents were frequently infected by *Coccidioides immitis* in regions where the disease was endemic but he finally concluded that infection of these animals was the result of their exposure to the same hazard of infection as man and the farm and domestic animals of the region.

Plants

Although probably every plant is susceptible to fungal infection and although fungi growing on plants or plant debris make a major contribution to the airspora involved in allergic conditions (see Chapter 7) plants appear to play a minor role as a reservoir of fungi pathogenic for man and animals. Gruby claimed to have infected an unnamed plant with the favus fungus (see Chapter 2) and Benham & Kesten (1932) succeeded in infecting carnations with *Sporothrix schenckii* which is believed to be transmitted to man by injury caused by thorns or prickly leaves as is the tropical mycetoma, the causal agents of which have been isolated from the thorns of desert plants.

One alleged case of human disease caused by an established plant-pathogenic fungus is the subcutaneous infection associated with *Cercospora apii*, which causes a leaf spot of celery, reported by Lie-Kian-Joe *et al.* in Indonesia in 1957. Others are the association of *Curvularia geniculata* with mycetoma in the dog (Bridges, 1957) and *Brachycladium spiciferum* [the *Drechslera* state of *Cochiobolus spicifera*] from nasal granulomas in cattle (Bridges, 1960), and mycetoma in the cat and a horse (Bridges & Beasley, 1960).

Mouldy hay is a source of the fungi causing mycotic placentitis and abortion in cattle and Austwick (1975) presented evidence that *Mortierella wolfii*, which is the main cause of this condition in New Zealand, originates from rotting silage of which the mould appears to be a secondary invader.

Weather

Attention has already been drawn to the association of outbreaks of coccidioidomycosis with summer dust storms in the United States where the incidence is highest during the warmer drier months. An interesting contribution to the epidemiology of sporotrichosis was made by Mackinnon (1948–9) who was able to ascertain the date of infection of 32 of a series of 46 cases of sporotrichosis which he studied in Uruguay between 1939 and 1948. Twenty-six patients were found to have contracted the disease in the autumn or early winter and in two years characterized by periods of heavy rain and high humidity small epidemics were noted at such times when, presumably, growth of the pathogen in its natural habitat was promoted and the chance of infection increased. An examination of the weather records of periods when epidemic infections occurred suggested that a relative humidity of 90% to saturation, a mean temperature of 16–20 °C with no low values at night, and abundant and repeated rainfall during a week or more were the required conditions and it was on this basis that Mackinnon claimed to have forecast the small outbreak of five cases that occurred in April 1947. In contrast to these results, González-Ochoa (1965) in Mexico found sporotrichosis to be associated with cooler times of the year.

Hugh-jones & Austwick (1967) found interesting correlations between rainfall and the incidence of bovine mycotic abortion as indicated by the number of infected placentae received during 1959 to 1966 at the Ministry of Agriculture, Fisheries & Food's Central Veterinary Laboratory from veterinary practices in the Weybridge Veterinary Investigation area. Clear statistical relationships were established. The number of days that it rained in June was directly correlated during the following twelve months with the mycotic abortion rate attributed to *Aspergillus* while the incidence of mucoraceous placental infections was inversely related to the number of rainy days in September. It was suggested that mouldy hay is the common source of the infection and that a wet main haymaking season allowed a heavy *Aspergillus* build up in the damp hay while a wet September resulted in a light, and a dry month in a heavy, cut of late hay in which the higher soluble carbohydrate content favours the growth of mucoraceous fungi. The incidence of farmer's lung (see Chapter 7) also shows a positive correlation with wet hay harvests.

A more firmly statistically based relationship of a mycosis with the weather was provided by L. P. Smith & Austwick (1975) who established a correlation between rainfall and the incidence of mycotic dermatitis ('lumpy wool') in sheep caused by the actinomycete *Dermatophilus congolensis*, as measured by the percentage of infection in a flock or the percentage of substandard ('cast') wool in the clip. Mycotic dermatitis, which has a worldwide distribution, is characterized by the formation of scabs which are carried away from the skin by growth of the wool and at the same time undergo changes in colour to give a zonation, and so a downgrading of the clip. Experimental studies suggested that the infection is spread by motile spores by a splash mechanism during heavy rain and the coarser the wool fibre the lower the percentage infection. It is believed that sheep infected during periods of heavy rain in one season spread the disease to others the following summer when there is heavy rain although in fine-woolled sheep epidemic spread may be built up in one summer. From observations on experimentally and naturally infected flocks (see Fig. 32) it was found that the best correlation was of infection with the number of occasions of heavy rain during the previous two years and it was concluded that 'with the aid of meteorological data it should be quite

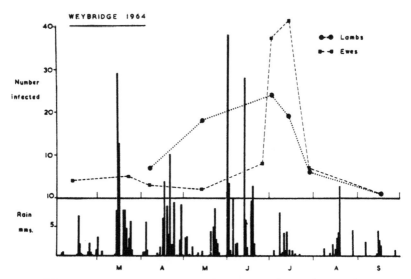

Figure 3.   Outbreaks of Dermatophilus infection
in lambs and ewes in relation to rainfall 1964.
Weybridge.

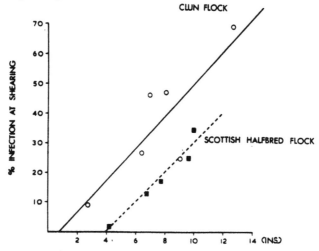

Figure 4.   Regression curves for infection
observed in May in Clun Forest and Scottish half-
bred flocks in relation to the cumulative rainfall for July, August and September of the previous
year.   Porton Down and Hurley.

Fig. 32. Relationship of dermatophilosis in sheep to the weather.
(Smith & Austwick, 1975, figs 3, 4).

feasible to produce forecasts of acceptable accuracy on the quality of the forthcoming wool clip some six months before shearing and grading takes place'.

4. The 'compromised' patient

The notion that mycoses are influenced or even caused by constitutional factors is one of long standing. As already noted (Chapter 4), even after the aetiology of ringworm had been established some refused to accept the infectious nature of the disease. Similarly, later in the nineteenth century the rôle of the pathogen in the aetiology of thrush was being questioned. Armand Trousseau [1801–67], a famous Parisian physician, whose opinion of 'micrographers' was low, while accepting that 'the characteristic element of thrush is a cryptogamic plant' considered it

'equally a matter of certainty that for the development of the mycelium, special conditions are requisite: there must be pre-existing inflammation of the mucous membrane on which it is seated...' (Trousseau, 1869:620).

Parrot (1877:88) was of the same opinion:

'...le muguet n'est pas une affection primordiale indépendante, mais que, toujours subordonné à un trouble functionel antérieur...'

Since then much evidence has accumulated that the incidence of certain mycoses depends on the age, sex, degree of immunity (whether inborn or acquired), or other abnormality, especially, during recent years, on iatrogenic factors to which the term 'compromised patient' has been particularly applied (see Warnock & Richardson, 1982). It has also become clear that some mycoses have to be included among occupational hazards, a topic reviewed by DiSalvo (1983).

The best known example of the effect of age is provided by classical tinea capitis of European children caused by *Microsporum audouinii* which if not cured by treatment usually resolves spontaneously at puberty possibly due to a change in the composition of the fatty acids secreted by the scalp. Rothman *et al.* (1947) isolated normal aliphatic monobasic acids with odd numbers of carbon acids (e.g. pelargonic and tridecanoic acids) from adult hair fat which although not killing the fungus spores within the hair prevent infection of new hair which replaces the old after shedding. This disease was exported from Europe into North America where it has become endemic but in tropical countries outbreaks are usually confined to children of European residents. Similarly, although tinea imbricata (*Trichophyton concentricum*) has not infrequently been recorded in Europe on individuals returning from the tropics it has never established itself in temperate regions.

An interesting observation on the effect of nutritional level on ringworm was that of the Dutch mycologist, the late M. A. Donk, on the incidence of mycotic skin infections among his fellow prisoners held captive in Java by the Japanese during the 1939–45 war as reported in Nickerson (1947:3):

Shortly after internment following the sharp break from high nutritional level to one of bare subsistence, the incidence of infections was high among the prisoners. As time went on and the weight of all decreased continuously, infections cleared and the incidence became quite low, reaching a vanishing point after three years internment, by which time most of the prisoners had lost up to half of their original weight. On liberation and the return of sufficient food, fungus infections flared dramatically among nearly all who had been confined, to disappear slowly as an individual gained weight over a period of time.

For coccidioidomycosis, although light- and dark-skinned races appear to be equally susceptible to the primary form it was early established that the latter are much more prone to the disseminated form and a fatal outcome. Unfortunately in California most of those employed in agriculture and so particularly exposed to the hazard of infection from the soil are coloured.

The many surveys that have been made on the incidence of yeasts (especially *Candida albicans*) in both healthy and diseased subjects have clearly shown many factors to be involved. In general, its seems that a higher proportion of hospital patients harbour yeasts than others. According to Odds (1979:54), who comprehensively reviews the whole topic, approximately 10% of normal subjects carry *C. albicans* in the mouth while the value for hospital patients is more than four times higher, the mean incidences for faeces being 14.6 and 22.0% respectively, for the two categories. Infancy and old age appear to favour candidosis and candida vaginitis tends to accompany pregnancy. Candida vaginitis, or other aspect of candidosis, is a frequent accompaniment of diabetes mellitus and cancer also has been claimed as a predisposing factor for mycotic infections (see Klastersky, 1982).

Since the introduction of penicillin and other antibacterial antibiotics evidence has often been presented to show that an increase in mycotic, particularly Candida, infection followed their use, presumably due to decreased competition for suitable substrata (e.g., Lehner & Ward (1970) at Guy's Hospital, London, reported the development of oral candidosis in patients treated with tetracycline or corticosteroids for oral ulcers.) This effect was probably real but records are complicated by an increase in both the intensity and accuracy in mycological diagnosis which occurred during the same period. That mycotic infection became an increasing hazard in open heart surgery, organ transplantation, and intravenous feeding has been well established. The first case of *Candida albicans* endocarditis following heart surgery was reported by Koelle and Pastor in 1956 from Philadelphia and there are many subsequent records,[10] infection originating during the many samplings for blood, from catheters, and the intravenous injection of therapeutants (which is sometimes due to prolonged treatment for bacterial endocarditis). Fungal endocarditis also occurs in drug addicts.

Candida is also the predominating fungal pathogen complicating organ transplantation as was revealed by the analysis of 107 cases of kidney transplantation by Rifkin *et al.* (1967), as it is in septicaemia associated with hyperalimentation when the portal of entry is most frequently the catheter (Vic-Dupont *et al.*, 1968).

Occupational hazards

The first association of mycotic infection with an occupation was that in France of pulmonary aspergillosis in 'faveurs de volailles' or 'gaveurs de pigeons' – squab feeders – who fattened young birds for the market by chewing grain in their own mouths and then forcing it into the gullets of the birds with their tongues (Dieulafoy *et al.*, 1890; Gaucher & Sergent, 1894), and Rénon (1895) recorded the same infection in the 'peigneurs de cheveux' who combed and sorted hair for wig making. Another example of a mycosis as an occupational hazard is provided by sporo-trichosis which is associated with gardening. An outbreak of sporotrichosis among florists has already been noted and Foerster (1926) reported the initiation of this mycosis by puncture of the skin by thorns of rose and barberry and that United States courts have been known to award compensation for the cost of medical care for sporotrichosis as an employment-connected disability. The high incidence of tinea pedis among those engaged in sport has long been recognized by the popular designation of the condition as 'athlete's foot' typically acquired from the floors of changing rooms and, particularly swimming baths as many surveys have shown (e.g. Gentles, 1956; English & Gibson, 1959; Drouhet *et al.*, 1967). Foot ringworm may also be considered an occupational disease of those in the armed services and also of coal miners among whom there have often been epidemic outbreaks following the introduction of pithead baths (Gentles & Holmes, 1957). Ringworm lesions on the hands and arms of laboratory animal attendants are also not infrequently the first indication of infections of the animals, such as that of *Trichophyton mentagrophytes* in mice which is inconspicuous.

5. Geographical distribution of mycoses

During the first quarter of the present century it was widely held that mycoses of both man and animals were characteristic of the tropics where fungi are more diverse and luxuriant than in temperate regions. The geographical distribution of the mycopathological literature gave little support for this notion. An analysis of the 750 references compiled in the bibliography of Sabouraud's *Les teignes*, 1910, shows 96% to have originated in Europe (43% in France). A similar analysis of the publications compiled in the *Review of Medical and Veterinary Mycology* for the years 1943–9 shows 61% have originated in North America 58% from the United States), 18% from Europe (4% from France); the values for Africa, Asia, and Australasia being 4, 2, and 1%, respectively. These statistics clearly reflect the distribution of mycologists and the intensity of their interest in mycoses rather than the distribution of fungi pathogenic for man and animals. Today, while the incidence of medical and veterinary mycologists, which is highest in the USA, still affects the recorded incidence and distribution of mycoses most regions of the world have been sufficiently well sampled to establish the geographical distribution of many mycoses.

Human actinomycosis has proved to be of worldwide distribution and, according to Cope (1938:27), has been diagnosed 'wherever there is a microscope and a laboratory'. Dermatophyte infections are equally wide-spread (see the reviews by Ajello (1960), Rippon (1982): 161–6) but the distribution of many species is more restricted. For example, *Trichophyton concentricum* (tinea imbricata) is endemic in the Far East and the Pacific region, *T. ferrugineum* in Japan, *T. simii* in India, while favus is caused by *T. schoenleinii* in western Europe but in north and central Africa and eastern Europe by *T. violaceum*. *Microsporum audouinii*, as already noted, originated in Europe and is now established in North America while the cat and dog Microsporum (*M. canis*) is sporadic and ubiquitous. Because of increased travel and its rapidity many dermatophytes have been recorded in western Europe and North America (where a high standard of diagnostic laboratory facilities prevails) outside their normal distribution but few ever become endemic, one exception being *T. rubrum*, a tropical species now well established throughout temperate regions.

Among systemic mycoses histoplasmosis (*Histoplasma capsulatum*), although most studied in the United States, has a worldwide distribution having been recorded from more than fifty countries, temperate and tropical, although its incidence is uneven and unaccountably low in western Europe. Coccidioidomycosis by contrast has a more restricted distribution in arid regions of the USA, Mexico, and South America; records of the disease in Russia and a few other countries being of doubtful validity. The distribution of blastomycosis (North American blastomycosis; *Blastomyces dermatitidis*) and paracoccidioidomycosis (South American blastomycosis; *Paracoccidioides brasiliensis*) is still in general that indicated by their former names. Paracoccidioidomycosis is restricted to Latin America from Mexico to Argentina and although blastomycosis is endemic in North America where it has been most studied, there are a few apparently autochthonous cases for Africa and elsewhere.

Histoplasmosis is interesting in having a geographic and clinically distinct variant associated particularly with tropical Africa. It was Duncan, in 1943 (see Duncan, 1947), who first differentiated this variant (from Ghana) in which the pathogen is characterized by larger yeast cells than those of normal *Histoplasma capsulatum*. Vanbreusegham observed the same condition from the Belgian Congo and in 1952 proposed a new species, *H. duboisii* (see Dubois *et al.*, 1952), although the current consensus is to follow Drouhet who awarded varietal status to the taxon in 1957.

6

Therapeutic problems

Over the centuries a multiplicity of remedies of diverse origins have been offered for the amelioration of disease in both man and animals. From earliest times to the end of the eighteenth century folklore and astrology had an important influence on the selection of animal, vegetable, and mineral products, ranging from dried vipers and human urine to powders of precious stones, prescribed by physicians, sometimes in elaborate formulations of up to two hundred or more ingredients. Pharmacopoeias of the seventeenth century attempted the compilation of the more reliable remedies but the *Pharmacopoeia Londonensis* (first published in 1618 by the Royal College of Physicians of London) of 1746 – although it excluded unicorn's horn and virgin's milk and the two famous antidotes for poisons, theriac and mithridatium (see Chapter 8), made their final appearance – still retained such medicaments as crabs' eyes and wood-lice. The mid-nineteenth century saw the initiation of several accelerating trends. Successive editions of pharmacopoeias and their supplements included fewer and fewer natural products which have been replaced by chemically defined active ingredients and increasing numbers of pure chemicals synthesized in the laboratory and given recognition after prolonged and successful clinical trials. Furthermore, formulations have been simplified, pills have been replaced by tablets, and solutions for injection incorporated. These developments have been accompanied by the introduction of laboratory techniques for determining the sensitivity of pathogens to particular drugs and the concentration of therapeutants in body fluids.

The therapy of mycotic infections has been subject to the same pattern but as up to the beginning of the nineteenth century only cutaneous infections (including infection of the mucosa) were known, the diversity of the remedies employed was much more limited. The recognition of actinomycosis and subcutaneous and systemic mycoses during the second half of the century and since led to the deployment of a number of new therapeutants, some of which also proved of service for cutaneous mycoses.

Superficial and cutaneous mycoses

Ringworm (especially favus) of the skin and hair and thrush of the mucosa have been recognized for two millenia (see Chapter 1) and recommendations for their treatment have been many. Celsus for thrush proposed that 'the child's ulcers are to be anointed with honey, to which is added shumach...'[1] (*De re medica*, Book vi (11)), and in the eighteenth century Rosén von Rosenstein (1776) was recommending as efficacious for the same purpose 'Mr Boyle's remedy' composed of equal parts of *Sempervivum majus* juice and honey to which, after boiling, alum was added to give it 'a slightly austere taste' – the aphthae being touched every hour with the preparation. A century later Trousseau (1869:627–8) prescribed borax or potassium chlorate and honey. In Sweden, thrush lichen or lichen moss (*Peltigera aphthosa*) boiled in milk was a folk cure for thrush.

Pliny, in *Historia naturalis*, wrote of ringworm:

Bears' grease, mixed with ladanum and the plant adiantum, prevents the hair falling out; it is a cure for alopecy... Used with wine it is good for the porrigo, a malady which is also treated with ashes of deer's horns in wine; this last substance also prevents the growth of vermin in the hair. For porrigo some persons employ goat's gall, in combination with Cimolian chalk and vinegar, leaving the preparation to dry for a time on the head. Sow's gall, too, mixed with bull's urine, is employed for a similar purpose (Book xxvii, ch. 47).[2]

And in another place:

Juice of garlic is sometimes injected into the ears with goose-grease, and, taken in drink, or similarly injected, in combination with vinegar and nitre, it arrests phthiriasis [lice infestation] and porrigo (Book xx, ch. 23).[3]

Among the many substances and preparations used before about 1950 for the topical treatment of human ringworm and pityriasis have been: sulphur (both elemental and liver of sulphur (sulphurated potash)), mercury (mercuric chloride (corrosive sublimate), ammoniated mercury, phenyl mercuric nitrate), copper (as sulphate, acetate, oleate, etc.), silver nitrate, aluminium chloride, antimony compounds, selenium sulphide, iodine (elemental and as iodides), potassium permanganate, and borax; and among organic compounds alcohol, acetic, propionic, capryllic, undecenoic, oleic, benzoic, and salicylic acids, salicylanilide, tannin, tar (as tar water and tar ointment), chrysarobin, podophyllin, and the dyes gentian violet and carbolfuchsin.

In veterinary practice similar remedies were used. For example, in the 1908 Leaflet for farmers on cattle ringworm of the Board of Agriculture

& Fisheries of England and Wales train oil, lard, or soft soap combined with sulphur, iodine, or copper oleate were the recommended treatments (for which mercury biniodide (HgI$_2$) was substituted in later revisions) and in the Leaflet on white comb (*Microsporum gallinae*) of poultry, silver nitrate in soft paraffin was the treatment of choice.

Little experimental testing for antifungal properties was undertaken but in June 1855 Küchenmeister made a comparison of some recommended remedies for ringworm against vegetable parasites. He divided a quantity of densely moulded pumper-nickel [black wholemeal rye bread] into a number of portions which he treated with *Tinct. Veratri albi* [an alcoholic extract of *Veratrum album* roots], aqueous solutions of copper acetate (1:100) and corrosive sublimate (1:500), *Aqua phaged* [*aenica*] *pharmacop-*[*oeia*] *Würtemberg* [a mercuric chloride preparation], concentrated watery solutions of tanin and borax, *Aqua creosoti*, *Aqua picis* [tar water], and *Unguetum picis*. Others were left untreated. He made observations after 1,4,6 and 10 days, repeating some treatments, and from the fourth day introduced treatment with 80° alcohol (also diluted) either alone or as a supplement to the original treatments. The tincture and the tar ointment treatments were completely successful on the areas to which they were applied; so too was alcohol. The aqueous solutions were ineffective. *Tinct. veratri albi* had long been in use against pityriasis which was not recognized as mycotic until 1846, by Eichstedt. Küchenmeister reported his results to Professor Hebra of Vienna with a request that the professor would test spirituous remedies against favus. In response Hebra treated two patients after epilation with an alcoholic solution of veratrum with satisfactory results (Küchenmeister, 1857:236–41, 258).

Two earlier remedies which have survived to the present day are Whitfield's ointment and Castellani's paint. The former which proved so popular and for long provided a standard against which other panaceas for ringworm were measured, originated as a result of an accidental laboratory infection of Whitfield's forearm. Treatment with iodine and carbolic acid having failed Whitfield 'then rubbed in an ointment of 5 per cent benzoic acid and 3 per cent salicylic acid in soft paraffin and coconut oil for three days and it disappeared'. He, therefore, ventured 'to recommend the use of the ointment for general use in superficial tinea' (Whitfield, 1912). The inspiration for Castellani's paint (or magenta paint), based on carbolfuschin (a triphenylmethane dye), devised by Castellani (1928) for the treatment of epidermophytosis of the toes ('mango toe') and still used for intertriginous infections may have been gentian violet[4] (chrystal violet, methyl violet; all triphenylmethane dyes) introduced a few years earlier for the treatment of superficial Candida infections (Faber & Dickey, 1925). This last became the standard for Candida paronychia (Gomez-Vega, 1935) and Candida vaginitis until replaced by nystatin, imidazoles, etc. (see below).

Epilation

From the end of the eighteenth century the importance of epilation in accelerating recovery from favus or other ringworm infection of the scalp became generally realized. Various short cuts to achieve this were devised. The oldest was the 'calotte' [skull cap] or 'Jew's nightcap'[5] by which the epilation of the entire scalp was attempted in a single operation by the application of a pitch plaster which was then, after a suitable interval, removed in one piece. This method fell into disuse because of its barbarity. Another method, apparently practised in Hebra's clinic in the mid-century, was for diseased children to tear one another's hair out which, as Küchenmeister comments, 'is, no doubt, very recommendable and saves time to the physician'. The usual procedure was manual epilation with the fingers, combs, or tweezers (the last were first used by Plumb, 1824) after the hairs had been loosened by the disease itself or inducing inflammation with croton oil or other treatment and the epidermis softened with a warm poultice of oil and rye flour; the hair having first been cut short and the head cleansed by soap and water. Manual epilation of a whole head (which in the case of favus might take a day) was tedious and 'very tiresome and harassing to the operator, who is often haunted by the disgusting sight for several days, in consequence of the strain on the eyes'.[6] Fungicidal applications were then routinely applied to the epilated head while the hair regrew.

During the closing years of the eighteen-nineties there was a breakthrough in the technique of epilation. In 1896 Freund and Schiff in Vienna observed the fall of hair from a *naevus pilosus* [hairy mole] treated by X-rays. The next year Sabouraud in Paris was consulted by a young woman for a complete loss of hair in the occipital region after she had taken part in a public demonstration at which a metal chain necklace under her dress was revealed on a fluorescent screen by X-rays. The hair regrew normally in four months. Sabouraud was at the time studying the epilatory effect of the administration of thallium acetate by mouth but like others he at once saw the potential of X-ray epilation and the exploitation of this potential is particularly associated with the names of Sabouraud and his collaborator Henri Noiré (Sabouraud & Noiré, 1904; Sabouraud,

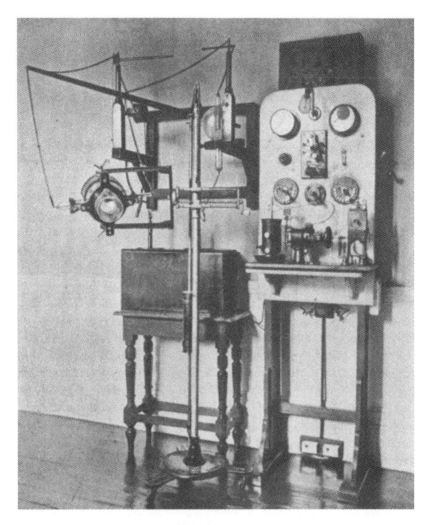

Fig. 33. X-ray apparatus for epilation used in London by J. M. H. Macleod. Now in the Wellcome Museum of the History of Medicine. (Macleod, *Diseases of the skin*, London, 1920, fig. 19).

1910:770–812) who had the misfortune to die from X-ray injury. Suitable apparatus for the routine treatment of children by X-rays at the St Louis Hospital was devised and a colorimetric method based on the change in colour of platinum cyanide-treated paper when exposed to X-rays was developed for controlling the dose because an overdose of radiation results in permanent baldness. An early X-ray apparatus for epilation (Fig. 33) used in London was that designed by A. L. Dean (who

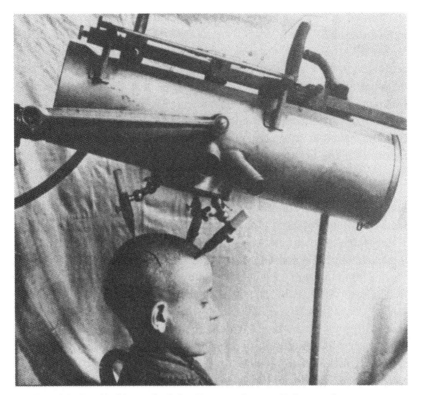

Fig. 34. Kienböck's method for X-ray epilation. (Sabouraud, 1910, fig. 433).

also died from X-ray injury) for the dermatologist J. E. M. Macleod after the latter visited Sabouraud's clinic in 1904.[7] In 1909, Adamson adapted a method devised by Kienbock in Vienna so that a scalp could be completely epilated by five applications of X-rays (directed at the front, crown, and back and the two sides of the head) so controlled that no area received a damaging dose of radiation. Accurate selection of the areas treated was assisted by a flat circular metal ring on the underside of which were three adjustable legs. This enabled the X-ray application to be made at right angles to the head with the X-ray source at a constant distance from the scalp (see Fig. 34).

At the beginning of the present century ringworm was a major problem in schools of London and other large cities. The disease is contagious, so isolation was indicated, and the treatment long and uncertain. In 1901 to obviate the educational disturbance the London Asylums Board started a special school where in succeeding years six hundred to a thousand children, of an estimated three thousand infected in the London area, were treated annually. The average length of treatment was nineteen months. From 1905 this period was dramatically reduced to four months after the introduction of X-ray epilation; the average cost per week per child, including maintenance, clothing, teaching, and treatment, being 13 shillings and 7 pence [£0.68] (Adamson, 1910; Shanks, 1967). X-ray epilation became general practice but where X-ray facilities were lacking thallium epilation was often resorted to when care had to be taken to ensure that the dose was correctly adjusted to body weight in order to avoid serious side effects.

Another major technical advance which greatly facilitated diagnosis of head ringworm in children was the discovery in 1925 by the French workers Margarot and Devèze that *Microsporum*-infected (but not *Trichophyton*-infected) hairs show a brilliant greenish fluorescence in ultraviolet light ('Wood's light') obtained by filtering light from a mercury vapour lamp through soda glass containing nickel oxide (as first described by Professor R. H. Wood of Johns Hopkins University) (see Margarot & Devèze, 1929; Kinnear, 1931). This technique greatly simplified diagnosis (especially in cats and dogs in which the signs are often very inconspicuous and the first indication of infection the development of ringworm in the animal's owner), the selection of hairs for microscopic and cultural examination, and the test for a cure. By the use of Wood's light and X-ray epilation head ringworm in the United Kingdom was reduced to a very low level during the years preceding 1939 but the disturbances in family life during the Second World War, crowded air raid shelters, and the evacuation of children from cities resulted in an increase in the disease which now has again been reduced to a low level. The way in which a public health organization tackled an outbreak by enlisting the co-operation of parents, school teachers, hairdressers, and the local cinema and by setting up local 'ringworm schools' is well illustrated by the account by Keddie (1947) of an outbreak of seven hundred cases in two towns in Scotland.

Epilation is no longer a routine procedure for tinea capitis because of the introduction of the antibiotic griseofulvin.

Griseofulvin

The exploitation of penicillin during the 1939–45 war stimulated searches for other antibiotics worldwide. These searches were either random or systematic and success depended largely on luck and the competence of the biochemical and clinical support. At first this search was mainly for

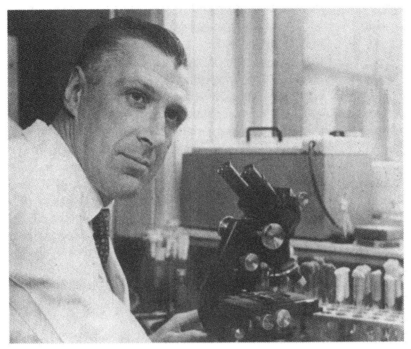

Fig. 35. J. C. Gentles who introduced griseofulvin therapy for ringworm.

antibiotics active against the tubercle bacillus and other bacteria unaffected by penicillin but the screening was later extended to cover many other micro-organisms, including fungi. Many antifungal antibiotics have been described but few have reached clinical practice because of instability, toxicity, or other objectionable side-effects. The three most important, all commercially available, have been nystatin, amphotericin B, and griseofulvin.

Griseofulvin, a chlorine-containing polyketide, was first described as a secondary metabolite of *Penicillium griseofulvum* by Oxford, Raistrick & Simonart (1939). Independently Brian, Curtis & Hemming (1946) reported what they called 'curling factor' from *P. janczewskii* [= *P. nigricans*] which distorted the growth of hyphal tips and the next year Grove and McGowan showed 'curling factor' to be identical with griseofulvin. Brian and his team demonstrated that griseofulvin could act as a systemic fungicide in plants and in 1958 J. C. Gentles (Fig. 35) of Glasgow University when seeking a systemic treatment for ringworm demonstrated the successful use of griseofulvin *per os* against experimental infections of *Microsporum canis* and *Trichophyton mentagrophytes* in guinea-pigs.[8] Shortly afterward Lauder & O'Sullivan (1958) of the University of Glasgow Veterinary School found that griseofulvin administered orally to calves prevented experimental infection by the cattle ringworm fungus (*T. verrucosum*) and cured established infections and Williams, Marten & Sarkany (1958) reported from King's College Hospital, London, promising results in the treatment of nine cases of *T. rubrum* infection of the skin and nails and one of *M. audouinii* infection by the administration of 0.5 g of griseofulvin four times a day. No side-effects were observed. This successful treatment of human ringworm was amply confirmed by hundreds of publications from all parts of the world and griseofulvin was the subject of an international symposium[9] and other meetings. The introduction of small-particle griseofulvin about 1965 allowed the total normal daily dose of 1 g to be halved. Griseofulvin was first marketed in the UK in the spring of 1959 by Glaxo (as Grisovin) and Imperial Chemical Industries (as Fulcin). The sales have been enormous. It was estimated that in the United States alone they totalled 6 million dollars for 1966.[10]

Nystatin A complementary antibiotic of equal importance for use against candidosis and other yeast infections was *nystatin*, a polyene (tetraene), first produced by a strain of *Streptomyces noursei* at the New York Branch Laboratory of the New York State Department of Health by the mycologist Elizabeth Hazen[11] (Fig. 36) from a sample of soil she had collected, while on holiday, on the farm of Walter B. Nourse in Virginia; developed in collaboration with a biochemist Rachael Brown[11] (Fig. 36) working at the New York City Central Laboratory, Albany; and named fungicidin (a name later changed to honour New York State). A patent application was filed by the Research Corporation (the New York foundation for the advancement of science) in 1951 and U.S. Patent 2 797 183 granted on 25 June 1957. E. R. Squibb & Sons were given exclusive right to manufacture and sell the antibiotic for five years. Between 1955 and 1976 (when the patent expired) the accruing royalties totalled 3.4 million dollars which were divided equally between the Research Corporation and the Brown-Hazen Fund specially created to support research and teaching in the medical and biological sciences, including medical mycology. Nystatin, particularly successful as a treatment for Candida infections whether superficial or deep-seated, is available in a variety of formulations. Although toxic when administered parenterally, nystatin can be given by mouth as it is not

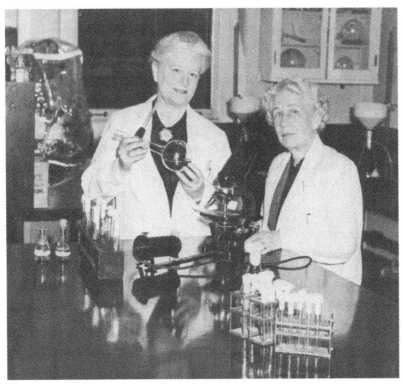

Fig. 36. Rachael F. Brown (1898–1980) (left) and Elizabeth L. Hazen (1885–1975) (right) who discovered nystatin.

absorbed by the gut. Side-effects are minimal and species of Candida do not readily acquire resistance to the drug.

Another antibiotic, discovered by Alma Whiffen (see Leach, Ford & Whiffen, 1947), which is familiar to mycopathologists, particularly those interested in ringworm, is *cyclohexamide* (Actidione), a water-soluble thermostable diketone from *Streptomyces griseus* which inhibits the growth of some yeasts (including *Cryptococcus neoformans* against which it found a therapeutic use before the introduction of amphotericin B) and some mycelial fungi. Its best known use is in combination with penicillin and streptomycin as an addition to the culture medium designed by Georg *et al.* (1954) for the selective isolation of dermatophytes and other pathogenic fungi.

Immunization

Although serological testing proved a valuable diagnostic technique for mycotic infections (see Chapter 5), immunization, apart from experimental studies on laboratory animals, has been little used against mycoses. One exception is the many reports from the USSR during the past decade and a half of the successful use of a vaccine against cattle ringworm. Up to 1975, the vaccine TF-130 (or LTF-130, the lyophilized version) prepared from *Trichophyton verrucosum* was used to immunize *c.* 90 million young cattle resulting, it was claimed, in a more than 90% reduction in the incidence of ringworm between 1968 and 1975 (Sarkisov, 1976).

Subcutaneous and systemic mycoses

It was probably the discovery by the Geneva physician Jean-François Coindet [1774–1834] which he announced to the Swiss Society of Natural Sciences on 25 July 1820 that iodine (known since 1813) was a specific for goitre that provided the inspiration for the use of iodine against actinomycosis (lumpy jaw) and actinobacillosis (wooden tongue) (see Chapter 1) in cattle (see Chapter 1) but who first introduced this therapy is still uncertain. Cope (1938) attributed the introduction to Professor H. J. P. Thomassen of Utrecht in 1885 but from a questionnaire to veterinarians distributed during the late eighteen-seventies by J. W. Axe, professor of pathology at the Royal Veterinary College, London, it appeared that the use of potassium iodide against these infections was already well established. William Dick, the famous Edinburgh veterinary surgeon, treated 'clyers' (actinomycosis) of cattle with iodine as early as 1839.[12] Potassium iodine administration (combined with surgery as necessary) became the standard treatment for actinomycosis (although only a specific for actinobacillosis) until replaced, or supplemented, about 1940, by sulphadiazine and other sulphonamides. A few years later these all gave way to penicillin therapy (Nichols & Herrell, 1948) to which both *Actinomyces* and *Nocardia* are sensitive.

Potassium iodine was first successfully used, at Sabouraud's suggestion, for sporotrichosis by de Beurmann & Ramond (1903) for which it is still the recommended treatment. Iodine has also been used, successfully, against aspergillosis, both avian and human, and, usually unsuccessfully, against many other mycoses (including dermatophyte infections) so that its use is now limited to sporotrichosis therapy.

During the nineteen-thirties and forties, and to a lesser extent today, sulphonamides were deployed against a range of systemic mycoses. Effort was then diverted to the search for new antibiotics – including antifungal antibiotics – and as already noted the major success was amphotericin.

Amphotericin B

Amphotericin B, another polyene (heptaene), produced by *Streptomyces nodosus*, was first reported by Gold *et al.* in 1956. Given orally or parenterally amphotericin B has proved its value against all the major systemic mycoses for which it has been the most used therapeutant in spite of irreversible nephrotoxic side-effects, the severity of which depend on the amount of the drug administered. It is also used topically for superficial infections.

Other polyenes from streptomycetes having antifungal properties and varying degrees of therapeutic potential include *candicidin* (from *Streptomyces griseus*; introduced in the USA, 1953),[13] *trichomycin* (*S. hachijoensis* and *S. abikoensis*; Japan, 1955)[14]; *filipin* (*S. filipinensis*; USA, 1955)[15]; *etruscomycin* (or lucenomycin; *S. lucensis*; Italy, 1957)[16]; *pimaricin* (or natamycin; *S. natalensis*; Netherlands, 1958)[17]; and *hamycin* (*S. pimprina*; India, 1961).[18]

In parallel to the search for antibiotics major pharmaceutical companies consistently attempted the discovery and development of new chemotherapeutants, including antifungal products. Chemists synthesized series of new organic compounds, based on structures thought most likely to yield positive results, which were then screened for activity against fungi and other pathogenic agents. Two successes for clinical use against fungi were flucytosine and the imidazoles.

Flucytosine

Flucytosine (5-fluorocytosine), first synthesized in 1957 as a potential cytostatic agent, was patented in 1962 by J. Berger and R. Duschinsky as an antifungal agent which proved itself clinically acceptable, particularly for septicaemic candidosis and cryptococcosis (but also useful in systemic aspergillosis and chromomycosis) for which it has provided an alternative (or synergic supplement; Bennett *et al.*, 1979) to amphotericin B which is more toxic to man than flucytosine.

Imidazoles

An important group of antifungal agents are the imidazoles, derivatives of benzimidazole which had been known since 1952 to yield antifungal derivatives. The first success was chlorobenzyl imidazole, *chlormidazole*, which was marketed by the Chemie Grünenthal GmbH from 1958 in formulations for use against cutaneous mycoses. In 1969 two other imidazoles were simultaneously made commercially available – *clotrimazole* ('Canesten'; *bis*-phenyl-(2-chloro-phenyl)-1-imidolylmethane) by Bayer AG in Germany and *miconazole* (1-2,4-dichloro-β-(2,4-dichlorobenzyloxy) phenethyl imidazole nitrate) by Janssen Pharmaceutica in Belgium – which have both become established because of their ability to inhibit the growth of all pathogenic fungi; miconazole is the drug of choice against *Pseudallescheria boydii* infections (Lutwick *et al.*, 1979).

Environmental manipulation

It is sometimes possible to control, or greatly reduce, the incidence of mycotic infection by adjusting the environment. Cattle ringworm, for example, is frequently most severe among calves. Spraying the walls and woodwork of the calf sheds with a fungicide reduces new infections and prevents the spores of the pathogen being carried over to the next season. Similarly, tinea pedis infections have been reduced by treating the floors of swimming baths and pit-head baths with fungicides.

During the 1945–9 war the incidence of coccidioidomycosis among troops stationed in the San Joaquin Valley of California was reduced by one third to a half by grassing air fields and spraying athletic grounds with mineral oil (Smith *et al.*, 1946). Likewise, treatment of the soil with formalin to eradicate *Histoplasma capsulatum* from endemic sites has been effective (Tosh *et al.*, 1967).

Again, in the largest outbreak of sporotrichosis ever recorded involving the infection during 1941–3, of 2825 workers in the Venterspost and Consolidated Main Reef gold mines of the Witwatersrand in South Africa, the main source of infection was the growth of the pathogen on the mine timbers under the conditions of high humidity which prevailed. Spraying the timbers with fungicides and bringing only new timber into the mines after treatment controlled the epidemic (see *Sporotrichosis...*, 1947).

In England, C. J. La Touche, after working as a mycologist for twenty years qualified in medicine. On taking a post in medical mycology at Leeds he attempted the eradication of small epidemic outbreaks of ringworm then frequent in that city among children and domestic animals. He organized a squad which visited the homes of affected children and examined all members of the family and the local cats and dogs under Wood's light for Microsporum infection. The children were appropriately treated and the source of infection eliminated, sometimes infected cats

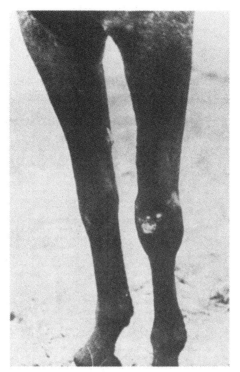

Fig. 37. Epizootic lymphangitis (*Histoplasma farciminosum*) in an Indian country-bred horse, extending from the knee (the original seat of infection) up fore-leg. (Pallin, 1904, plate vii).

being taken to the laboratory and therapy attempted. During 1950–4, 146 human infections were found in family groups totalling 226 individuals. Twenty-nine infections in cats and in dogs were also recorded (La Touche, 1952, 1955).

Legislation

Today, throughout the world certain diseases of man, animals, and plants are subject to legislation in efforts to prevent their introduction or spread, or effect their eradication. The first legislation to be promulgated against a fungus disease of animals was that enacted against epizootic lymphangitis of horses, asses, and mules. This mycosis, caused by *Histoplasma farciminosum* and characterized by suppuration of the superficial and subcutaneous lymphatic vessels (Fig. 37), was for long confused with glanders (farcy) and ulcerative lymphangitis and it has a wide distribution from Europe and North Africa to India and Sri Lanka. The disease which

(5664.)

ORDER OF THE MINISTER OF AGRICULTURE
AND FISHERIES.

(*Dated 3rd March,* 1938.)

EPIZOOTIC LYMPHANGITIS ORDER OF 1938.

The Minister of Agriculture and Fisheries, by virtue and in exercise of the powers vested in him under the Diseases of Animals Acts, 1894 to 1937, and the Agriculture Act, 1937, and of every other power enabling him in this behalf, hereby orders as follows:—

Notice of Disease.

1.—(1) Every person having or having had in his possession or under his charge any animal affected with or suspected of being affected with Epizootic Lymphangitis, or the carcase of such an animal shall (*a*) as far as practicable keep that animal or carcase separate from horses, asses, or mules not so affected or suspected; and (*b*) with all practicable speed give notice of the fact to a constable of the police force for the police area wherein the animal or carcase is or was.

(2) A veterinary surgeon who examines any animal or carcase and is of opinion that the animal is affected with Epizootic Lymphangitis, or was so affected when it died or was slaughtered, or suspects the existence of that disease therein, shall with all practicable speed give notice of the existence or suspected existence of the disease to a constable of the police force for the police area wherein the animal or carcase is.

(3) A constable receiving any such notice as aforesaid shall forthwith by the most expeditious means give information of the receipt by him of the notice to the Veterinary Inspector appointed for the time being by the Minister to receive such information within the area wherein the animal or carcase is, and also to an Inspector of the Local Authority, and the constable shall also transmit the information to the Ministry by telegram.*

(4) An Inspector of the Local Authority who receives information of the existence or suspected existence of the said disease shall forthwith report the same to the Local Authority.

(5) Where the notice of disease relates to a carcase of an animal that has died or been slaughtered in the District of a Local Authority other than the Local Authority which receives the notice, the latter shall forthwith inform the other Local Authority of the receipt of the notice.

(6) A veterinary surgeon who under and in accordance with this Order gives notice of the existence or suspected existence of the said disease shall be entitled to receive from the Minister

* The telegram should be addressed " Agrifi, Parl, London."

Fig. 38. Epizootic Lymphangitis Order.

had a limited distribution in South Africa around the ports was re-introduced into that country during the Boer war (1899–1902). From there it was imported by army horses into England where the first case was detected at Aldershot in 1902 and the following year it was reported from Ireland. These outbreaks caused much alarm. In January 1904 the Board of Agriculture & Fisheries circularized Local Authorities in Great Britain under the Diseases of Animals Acts of 1894–1903 alerting them to the danger. This was followed in April 1904 by the 'Epizootic Lymphangitis Order of 1904' which required every person having in his possession a horse affected with, or suspected of, epizootic lymphangitis to isolate the animal and with all possible speed inform a constable of the police (Fig.

38). A similar circular and a parallel Order were distributed and enacted in Ireland by the Department of Agriculture & Technical Instruction in March and May, respectively, 1904.[19] This prompt action and a slaughter policy successfully eliminated epizootic lymphangitis from the British Isles within two years.

7

Spores as allergens: a problem of sensitization

The floating matter of the air

Investigation of what Tyndall in 1881 called 'the floating matter of the air' (the 'air spora' of Gregory, 1952) began in connection with the problems of putrefaction, contagion, and spontaneous generation and various sampling techniques were used in diverse situations. In the winter of 1748–9 the Berlin botanist J. G. Gleditsch [1714–86] baited the air by putting sterile pieces of ripe melon in previously sterilized vessels, covering the mouths of the vessels with muslin, and setting them in various positions in his home and garden when mould developed on most of the pieces. C. G. Ehrenberg [1795–1876] (also of Berlin) in a long series of observations between 1830 and 1847 examined thousands of raindrops, snowflakes, and dewdrops for micro-organisms as well as specimens of dust from Germany, Switzerland, Egypt, the Himalayas, and elsewhere. He also made observations on dust deposits in various buildings including hospitals filled with severe cases of cholera. In 1846 in England, Angus Smith examined water condensed from breath and on windows for microbes and also solid impurities in the air of mines. He obtained some samples by filtering the air through cotton wool and in 1866, in connexion with experiments on disinfection for the Royal Commission on the Cattle Plague, obtained others by the agitation of a large volume of air with pure water in a stoppered bottle. Dr Dundas Thompson sampled the air of cholera wards by aspiration through Woulfe's bottles containing distilled water. Pasteur (1861) adopted the filtration technique but instead of cotton wool used a plug of gun-cotton (a nitro-cellulose) which could then be dissolved in an alcohol-ether mixture leaving the catch for microscopical examination. He found that the size of the catch varied with the site and that still air, such as that of the cellars of the Paris Observatory, contained few germs. (Tyndall demonstrated the same effect by showing that particles settled out of still air so that a beam of bright light passed through it became invisible.)

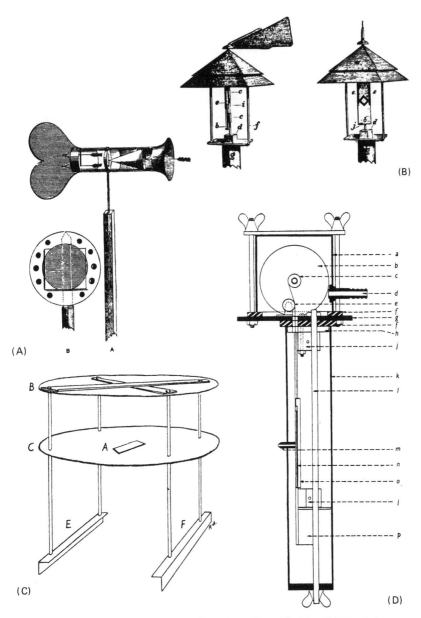

Fig. 39. Spore traps. A, Cunningham (1873); B, Blackley (1873, plate
v; side and front views); C, Hyde & Williams' device for exposing
gravity slides (H. A. Hyde & D. A. Williams, *New Phytologist* **43**, 43:
49, fig. 1, 1944); D, Hirst's volumetric spore trap (Hirst, 1952, text-fig.
1); m, orifice; n, slide; d, outlet tube.

During the London cholera epidemic of 1854 the Rev. Lord Godolphin Osborne exposed slips of glass, smeared with glycerin, to the air over cesspools, gully-holes, etc. near houses in which the disease appeared and 'caught what he termed "aerozoa", chiefly minute germs and spores of fungi'. Subsequently in America in 1862 J. H. Salisbury of Newark, Ohio, suspended pieces of glass overnight over pools and swamps and examined the drops of water found adhering to their undersides in his studies on the epidemiology of malaria which occurred in the marshy valleys of the Ohio and Mississippi rivers (Salisbury, 1866).

The method of sampling the air by impaction by gravity, air currents, wind, or applied suction proved the most fruitful. M. F. Pouchet[1], in France, developed what he called an 'aeroscope' which was the basis of R. L. Maddox's 'aeroconiscope' in England[2], a modified version of which (Fig. 39, A) was used by Cunningham in India (see below). Many other types of spore trap have been used (see Fig. 39). Most gave only qualitative information about the air spora but in the currently widely used 'Hirst trap' (developed by Hirst (1952) from May's 'cascade impactor'[3]) the air spora is continuously sampled and quantified by means of suction applied by an electric pump and a moving glass slide (Fig. 39, D). Another development which greatly helped the elucidation of many problems relating to the dispersal of spores was the construction by P. H. Gregory (1951), at Rothamsted Experimental Station, of a small experimental wind tunnel which is still in use after more than thirty years of service.

A convincing early demonstration of the prevalence of fungus spores in the air was that by D. D. Cunningham, a surgeon of the Indian Medical Service on special duty attached to the Government's Sanitary Commission, who had been introduced to mycology by Berkeley, Hallier, and de Bary. Between March and September 1872, Cunningham tried to establish a correlation between the air spora and the incidence of diarrhoea, dysentery, cholera, ague, and dengue in the Presidency and Alipore Jails in Calcutta. He found no correlation, but on 59 occasions took 24-h samples at weekly intervals of the air spora with his 'aeroscope' and for each sampling published drawings of the catch (Cunningham, 1873) (Fig. 40).

From 1875 routine sampling of the air for dust, bacteria, mould, spores, etc. was undertaken at the Observatoire Montsouris in the Parc Montsouris situated in the southern outskirts of Paris. This study is particularly associated with the name of the bacteriologist Pierre Miquel [1850–1922] who was in charge of the work for 34 years and who is still remembered for his doctoral thesis *Les organismes vivant de l'atmosphère*, 1883, and for the quantitative techniques he developed for estimating the air spora.

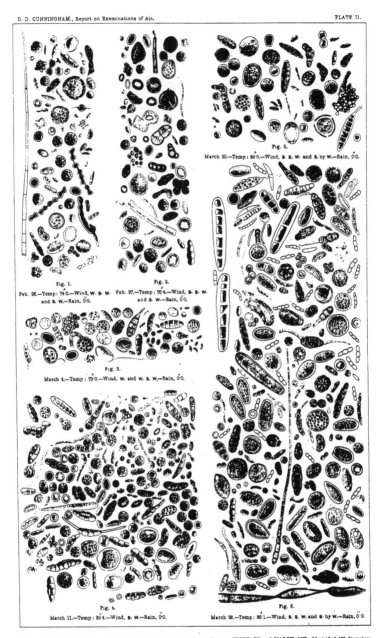

Fig. 5.

March 20.—Temp: 84·0.—Wind, s. s. w. and s. by w.—Rain, 0·0.

Fig. 1.

Feb. 26.—Temp: 74·0.—Wind, w. s. w. and s. w.—Rain, 0·0.

Fig. 2.

Feb. 27.—Temp: 76·4.—Wind, s. s. w. and s. w.—Rain, 0·0.

Fig. 3.

March 4.—Temp : 79·0.—Wind, w. and w. s. w.—Rain, 0·0.

Fig. 4.

March 11.—Temp : 82·4.—Wind, s. w.—Rain, 0·0.

Fig. 6.

March 28.—Temp: 86·1.—Wind, s. s. w. and s· by w.—Rain, 0·0.

ATMOSPHERIC ORGANISMS, &c. Collected During Periods of Twenty-four Hours in FEBRUARY and MARCH, 1872; Magnified 400 diameters.

(ALIPORE.)

Fig. 40. Spore catches collected during periods of 24 h in February and March, 1872, at Alipore. (Cunningham, 1873, plate, ii.)

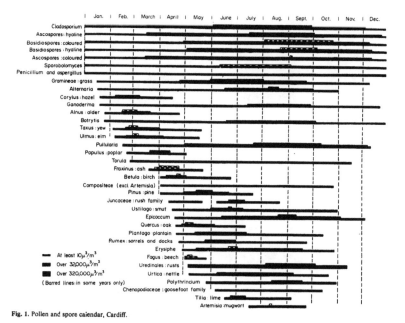

Fig. 1. Pollen and spore calendar, Cardiff.

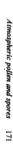

Fig. 41. Seasonal distribution of fungus spores (and pollen) at Cardiff. (Hyde, 1972, fig. 1).

Similar work was done concurrently in Berlin by the bacteriologist Walter Hesse [1846–1911], whose wife first suggested the use of agar-agar in place of gelatin in culture media.

Much is now known about the spores present in the air from ground level to the upper atmosphere as a result of the air sampling over both land and oceans in many parts of the world (see Gregory, 1973). These studies have shown fungus spores to be normally present in the atmosphere, often in large numbers. The pollen content of the air is naturally closely correlated with the season. Seasonal correlation is less marked for fungus spores (Fig. 41) although in the north temperate regions there is a well defined maximum spore content in the autumn and minimum during the winter months. Counts are particularly low after snow. Wet weather, which greatly reduces the number of dust particles, tends to increase the number of fungal spores and heavy rain may achieve only a temporary reduction. Another factor is the wind which is an important determinant of 'spore storms'. One of the most impressive and well documented of these storms occurred on 6–7 October 1937 throughout the eastern United States when, according to Durham (1938), the weather records showed that air masses from the north-west at an altitude of 2 000–6 000 feet moved rapidly east and south-east traversing Minnesota to the Atlantic seaboard in about 55 h. During this time thousands of tons of mould spores were transported several hundred miles. At nearly every station east of the Mississippi river the catch of *Alternaria* spores (up to 2 027 per 1.8 cm^2 per 24 h) was the highest of the year. At 17 of the stations the average increase in spore count was a hundred times that of the daily mean for October. Mass movements of cereal rust spores regularly occur in parts of North America, and India, and from North Africa to Europe where they are responsible for initiating outbreaks of cereal rust. The spore content of indoor air is normally lower than that of outdoor air but the former may attain exceptionally high values in cow sheds or other dusty situations.

The list of identified species recorded from air is long and the list of unidentified species even longer. In North America much attention has been paid to the incidence of *Alternaria* spores. This is partly because of the ease with which *Alternaria* spores can be recognized but evidence suggests that spores of this genus, which often predominate in that region where much land is devoted to cereals, are particularly important as allergens. *Alternaria* spores regularly occur in the air of the British Isles but in smaller numbers, the most numerous spores being those of *Cladosporium*, a genus which includes ubiquitous saprobic moulds. At the Asthma & Allergy Research Unit at St David's Hospital, Cardiff, where from the early nineteen-forties H. A. Hyde and D. A. Williams made long-term investigations of atmospheric pollen and fungus spores in relation to allergy[4], in 1948 *Cladosporium* colonies accounted for half of those developing on air plates and similar results have been obtained at other localities in the United Kingdom and elsewhere.

Fungi as allergens

The first published record of an allergic reaction to fungi is possibly that 'of a remarkable instance in Bonetus', referred to by Sir John Floyer in *A treatise of the asthma*, 1698 (p. 74), 'of an asthmatic who fell into a violent fit, by going into a wine cellar, where the must was fermenting...'. In 1700 Bernardino Ramazzini in his *De morbis diatriba*, the first book on occupational diseases, devoted Chapter XXVII to the diseases of 'the Sifters and Meters of Corn' where he wrote, in the words of the anonymous English translation of 1705 (pp. 171–2):

All Grain, and especially Wheat, whether kept in Pits under Ground, as in Tuscany, or in Barns, as in Countries upon the Po, have always a very small Powder mix'd with 'em; I mean not only that which they gather upon the Barn Floor in threshing, but another worse sort of Dust that Grain is apt to throw from itself upon long keeping. For the Seeds of Corn being replenish'd with a volatile Salt, insomuch that if they are not well dry'd in the Sun before they are laid up, they heat mightily, and turn presently to a Powder; it cannot but be that some thin Particles must flie off from the Husk that surrounds 'em, over and above the Powder and rotted Dust proceeding from the Consumption made by Moths, Worms, Mites, &c and Exrements. Now their being a Necessity of Sifting and Meting Corn and other Grain, the Men imploy'd in that Service are so plagu'd with this Powder or Dust, that when the Work is done they curse their Trade with a Thousand Imprecations. The Throat, the Lungs, and the Eyes sustain no small Damage by it, for it stuffs and dries up the Throat; it lines the Pulmonary Vessels with dusty Matter that causes a dry and obstinate Cough; and it makes the Eyes red and Watery. Hence it is that a'most all who live by that Trade, are short Breath'd, and Cachetick, and seldom live to be old; nay they are very apt to be sies'd with Orthopnoea, and last with Dropsie. Besides, this Powder has such a sharpness in it, that it causes violent itching, all over the Body.

Commenting on this syndrome, which has many features in common with farmer's lung associated with mouldy hay (see below), Ramazzini perceptively speculated on a possible connexion between the grain dust and the 'little worms' – bacteria – recently described by Leeuwenhoek.

Similar distress in farm workers and others after handling, or coming into contact with, mouldy straw was reported in Ohio by J. H. Salisbury (1862 a,b) who attempted to verify his clinical findings by dermal testing with spore suspensions from the affected straw, a procedure which consistently gave positive results of varying degrees of severity in the patients tested.

Although much attention was paid to the microscopic content of the air it was not until the mid-nineteenth century that experimental evidence was offered, by Charles Blackley, demonstrating allergy induced by fungus spores. Blackley, a Manchester physician, suffered from hay fever and made a prolonged study of his own condition, the results of which he published in a book, *Experimental researches on the causes and nature of catarrhus aestivus (hay-fever or hay-asthma)*, 1873, which is now a medical classic. He trapped pollen (Fig. 39, B) and tested the effects of inhaling pollen and a range of other agents, including fungi of which he wrote (pp. 57–8):

I had noticed many years ago that dust from straw sometimes brought on attacks of sneezing with me, and that this seemed to occur more frequently when we had had a long spell of wet weather. I determined to try what fungi could be generated on damp straw. For this purpose wheat straw, slightly moistened, was placed in a closed vessel, and kept at a temperature of 100° Fahr. In about twenty-four hours a small quantity of white mycelium was seen...This, I found on examination, was the *Penicillium glaucum*. After a few days another crop of dark-coloured spots were seen...These I found to be the *bristle mould* (*Chaetomium elatum*).

The spores of these two fungi were sown again separately on straw which had been placed in separate vessels having been subjected to the action of boiling water for a short time. A separate crop of each fungus was thus obtained.

The *odour* of the *Penicillium* produced no perceptible effect upon me, but the odour of the *Chaetomium* brought on nausea, faintness, and giddiness on two separate occasions. By inhaling the spores of the Penicillium...a severe attack of hoarseness, going on to complete aphonia, was brought on. This lasted for a couple of days, and ended in a sharpish attack of bronchial catarrh, which almost unfitted me for duty for a day or two...The sensations caused by these two agents were so unpleasant that I have never cared to reproduce them.

Mould asthma

The history of attempts to correlate the incidence of asthma with season, climate, altitude, and fungus spores has been summarized and documented by Van der Werf (1958). Only during the last fifty years has the importance of mould allergy been generally recognized. Outstanding among early workers was W. Storm van Leeuwen whose investigations[5] in the Netherlands into bronchial asthma, hay fever, and related conditions did much to stimulate others both in Europe and North America including A. W. Frankland of St Mary's Hospital Medical School, London, who appointed a mycologist (C. J. La Touche) to prepare mould antigens and investigate the moulds present in the homes of asthmatics, and S. M. Feinberg (1935, 1947) in the United States. It was in 1924 that Storm van Leeuwen noted in the island of Zuid-Beveland that 0.5 to 1.0% of the inhabitants of some villages were asthmatic, an incidence greatly in excess of that prevailing in other parts of the Netherlands. He failed to associate this condition with any meteorological peculiarity and attributed the cause to 'miasmata' or 'climate allergens'. Further, he showed that sufferers were relieved by air freed from 'miasmatic substances' by filtration through cotton wool or by passage through glycerin and he suggested that these airborne substances were mainly of fungus origin. He also found that high altitude gave relief and that inhaling dust from their homes provoked an attack of asthma. It was also in 1924 that Cadam in Canada recorded three cases of agricultural workers who developed severe asthma on exposure to dust from rusted grain and infected straw. He considered the stem rust (*Puccinia graminis*) to be the causal agent and he was able to induce a paroxysm by the inhalation of a few rust spores. According to Feinberg (1947), it is possible that the rust spores were contaminated with *Alternaria* or *Cladosporium* spores because spores of most rusts are ineffective as allergens and are obtained free from other spores with difficulty. Whether this was so or not Cadam was able to afford some relief with a vaccine prepared from the rust. In 1930, in the USA, Bernton described a case of asthma associated with *Aspergillus fumigatus*. Hopkins, Benham and Kesten in the same year described a similar case caused by *Alternaria* spores derived from vegetables stored in the basement of the patient's house and Durham (1938) stated that after the storm of *Alternaria* spores referred to above 'a brief inquiry has disclosed the correlation of clinical symptoms with the advent of the storm in some of the places affected'. Cobe (1932) described a case of asthma due to tomato leaf mould (*Fulvia fulva*), the spores of which occur in high concentrations in glasshouses containing affected plants and similar cases were cited by Brown (1936) and Morrow & Lowe (1943) while Frankland & Hay (1951) reported allergy caused by spores of the dry rot fungus (*Serpula lacrimans*) and Strand *et al.* (1967) two cases of 'lycoperdonosis', one in a boy who inhaled spores of a puffball (*Lycoperdon sp.*) in an attempt to control nose-bleeding, puffball spores being traditionally used to arrest bleeding.[6]

Kern (1921) was the first to obtain positive skin reactions with house dust extracts and the next year R. A. Cooke described a similar case of a patient who gave a strong skin reaction and developed mild asthma from an extract of the dust of his own room but not other allergens. The identity of the active fraction was not established but Cooke found that 109 (or 33%) of 327 asthmatic patients gave a positive reaction to 'dust'. A low percentage of normal people react to extracts of dust and the quite extensive literature on the antigenic properties of dust is somewhat conflicting. Moulds, if certainly one of the antigenic constituents of dust, are not the only one and are of less importance than, for example, mites (*Dermatophagoides*).

Farmer's lung

Some early records of farmer's, thresher's, or harvester's lung have already been referred to. Recent interest in this syndrome may be considered to have begun when Campbell (1932) reported five cases of acute respiratory symptoms following work with hay in Cumberland. Additional cases were subsequently reported from England, North America, and Scandinavia but in 1982 Eliasson noted that the condition has been well known in Iceland since 1790 when Dr Sveinn Palsson, a country physician, in an article on Icelandic disease nomenclature stated that:

Heysott [hay sickness] is the name of a disease of those who work with badly harvested and mouldy hay in winter. This is a well-known disease in Iceland, caused by the phlogistic vapours of the hay that are inhaled, leading to cold, fever, hoarseness, cough...[7]

Other Icelandic observations made between 1794 and 1913 cited by Eliasson showed that the allergic nature of the disease was understood and that a patient suffering from *heymaedi* [literally 'hay shortness of breath'], the modern Icelandic name for the condition, improved when no longer exposed to mouldy hay dust and that medicine had very little effect on the cure. It was also observed that heymaedi occurred in horses.

In England and elsewhere there was much speculation on the cause of the disease and a number of attempts made to elucidate its aetiology. F. Fawcett in 1936 considered it to be a mycosis ('bronchomycosis feniseciorum')[8] but J. T. Duncan was not impressed by this hypothesis. E. Törnell, ten years later, categorized it as a form of moniliasis [candidosis].[9] C. J. Fuller (1953) of the Royal Devon & Exeter Hospital in the light of a series of his own cases in the west of England favoured an allergic explanation and there were unsuccessful attempts to implicate particular fungal spores. Elucidation of the problem finally resulted from the collaboration of aerobiologists at Rothamsted Experimental Station and members of the Medical Research Council Research Group in Clinical Immunology at the Brompton Hospital in London (Pepys *et al.*, 1963). Gregory at Rothamsted put samples of mouldy hay associated with cases of farmer's lung in a wind tunnel and trapped the air-borne spores. It was soon established that certain aerobic thermophilic actinomycetes – particularly *Thermopolyspora polyspora* and *Micromonospora vulgaris* (which were later more correctly classified as *Micropolyspora faeni* (Cross *et al.*, 1968) and *Thermoactinomyces vulgaris*, respectively) – induced the formation of the 'farmer's lung hay' (FLH) antigen found in mouldy hay in normal hay, and *M. faeni* also in pure culture on artificial media. FLH antigen did not develop in hay after inoculation with fungi only or with any of six other actinomycetes tested and gave positive results in agar-gel double-diffusion immunoelectrophoresis tests against sera from patients with farmer's lung. Further, inhalation of an extract of *M. faeni* by affected subjects produced features of farmer's lung.

Typical *fog fever* in cattle is a respiratory disease of animals fed on aftermath ('foggage') during the autumn in the west of England but the name had also been applied to similar diseases, also of unknown aetiology, of housed cattle. Precipitins to FLH antigen were detected in the sera from the latter and Lacey (1968) found that the hay associated with such cases was rich in *M. faeni* and *T. vulgaris*. Pirie *et al.* (1971) claimed to have recorded the first confirmed case of farmer's lung in a cow.

In 1971 Lacey reported the association of *bagassosis* – a form of extrinsic allergic alveolitis in man induced by inhaling dust from mouldy, self-heated crushed sugar cane (bagasse) – with a new species of Thermoactinomyces (*T. sacchari*) and, in smaller quantities, *T. vulgaris* isolated from bagasse. Antigens from both actinomycetes gave positive precipitin reactions with sera from bagassosis patients.

Micropolyspora faeni and other thermophilic actinomycetes (as well as various fungus spores) have been associated frequently with 'humidifier fever' which has been widely reported during recent years associated with contaminated humidifiers in both commercial premises and private houses (see Edwards, 1977).

Occupational mould allergies

A number of other mould allergies have been established. Most, like farmer's lung, are occupational hazards. In 1848 Tersáncky drew attention to severe respiratory and dermal symptoms in workers engaged in the manufacture of tinder from polypores (*Fomes fomentarius, F. igniarius*) which had become very mouldy in store waiting to be processed. Hirt (1871) described the same phenomenon.

Michel (1863) described the 'mal de canne de Provence' (or 'cane cutter's disease') among reed cutters exposed to mouldy reeds (*Arundo donax*) which also became prevalent in the paper mills of the Midi of France where *Arundo donax* was being used for its fibre. The disease presented as lassitude, stiffness, low fever, and slight scrotal swelling. Later a prurigenous erythema spreads upwards from the inner surface of the thighs and becomes particularly severe in the armpits. A cough develops. Work is no longer possible. The patient is obliged to rest. His condition at once improves and recovery is complete in ten to fifteen days. On re-exposure to the reeds, symptoms recur. The condition was carefully investigated by Duché (1944) who attributed the complaint to the response of a sensitized individual to *Coniosporium arundinis* [*Papularia arundinis*, the *Arthrinium* state of *Apiospora montagnei*] which occurs on the lower leaves of reeds more than one year old.

'Maple-bark disease' (or 'maple-bark stripper's lung') which was first described by Towey *et al.* (1932) in Michigan and since reported elsewhere in North America (Emanuel *et al.*, 1966) is a rather similar condition caused by *Cryptostroma corticale* (syn. *Conisporium corticale*) which forms sheets of spores under the bark of both stored logs and growing trees.

Other mould allergies include 'cheese washer's lung' (attributed to the spores of *Penicillium casei*; Schlueter, 1973) in Switzerland among those who remove the mould from the outside of mature cheese, 'malster's lung' (*Aspergillus clavatus*) in Scotland (Blyth *et al.*, 1977) and elsewhere, 'suberosis' (associated with *Penicillium frequentans*) of workers in cork-making factories in Portugal (see Lacey, 1973), and 'mushroom worker's lung'.

8

Mycetism, mycotoxicoses, and
hallucinogenic fungi:
toxicological problems

1. Mycetism

That some of the larger fungi are poisonous to man has been on continual
record since Euripides [5th cent. BC], according to Eparchides, when on a
visit to Icarus composed an epigram to commemorate the death, on one
day, of a woman, her unmarried daughter, and two full-grown sons after
eating poisonous fungi gathered from the fields.[1] Typical of classical
references to fungi is that by the physician, grammarian, and poet
Nicander [c. 185 BC] in his six hundred line hexameter poem *Alexipharmaca*
on poisons and their antidotes:

Let not the evil ferment of the earth, which often causes swellings of the belly or
strictures in his throat, distress a man; for when it grows up under the viper's deep
hollow track it gives forth the poison and hard breathing of its mouth; an evil
ferment is that; men generally call the ferment by the name of fungus (μύκης),
but different kinds are distinguished by different names; but do thou take the
many-coated heads of the cabbage, or cut from around the twisting stems of the
rue or old copper particles which have long accumulated, or pound clematis into
dust with vinegar, then bruise the roots of pyrethrum, adding a sprinkling of
vinegar or soda, and the leaf of cress which grows in gardens, with the medic plant
and pungent mustard, and burn wine-lees into ashes or the dung of the domestic
fowl; then, putting your right finger in your throat to make you sick, vomit forth
the baneful pest.[2]

Pliny Secundus [c. AD 23/24–79] in his *Naturalis historia* commended
the edible *boleti* [gilled fungi, especially *Amanita caesarea*] but, like
Dioscorides [fl. AD 41–68] warned:

Noxious kinds must be entirely condemned; for if there be near them a hobnail
('caligaris clavus') or a bit of rusty iron or a piece of rotten cloth, forthwith the
plant, as it grows, elaborates the foreign juice and flavour into poison; and to
discern the different kinds country-folk and those who gather them are alone able.
Moreover they imbibe other noxious qualities besides; if, for instance, the hole of
a venomous serpent be near, and the serpent breathe upon them as they open,

116

because, from their natural affinity with poisonous substances, they are readily disposed to imbibe such poison. Therefore one must notice the time before the serpents have retired into their holes...(*Nat. hist.* xxii.22).[3]

Attempts were also made to offer generalizations for distinguishing edible from poisonous fungi. Diphilus, a physician who lived about the beginning of the third century BC, in his book, *Diet suitable for persons in good and bad health*, wrote of fungi:

...the wholesome kinds appear to be those which are easily peeled, are smooth and readily broken, such as grow on elms and pines; the unwholesome kinds are black, livid, and hard, and such as remain hard after boiling; such when eaten produce deadly effects.

And as an antidote he recommended:

...a draught of honey and water, or honey and vinegar, or soda and vinegar; after the draught the patient should vomit.[4]

The use of honey and water ('hydromel') as an antidote for fungus poisoning was first mentioned in the Corpus Hippocraticum, *Epidemics* vii, 102 [4th cent. BC], where it is recorded that:

Having eaten a raw fungus (*mukēs*), the daughter of Pausanias was seized with nausea (*asē*), suffocation (*pnigmos*), and pain in the stomach (*odunē gastros*). She was given hydromel to drink and was put in a hot bath, whereupon she vomited up the fungus; as the malady passed off, she perspired profusely.[5]

Pliny also expressed the view that fungi remaining hard after cooking are injurious and stated that 'All poisonous fungi have a livid colour' while the opinion of Horace [65–8 BC], 'Pratensibus optima fungis matura est; aliis male creditur' ('Fungi which grow in meadows are the best; it is not well to trust others')[6], is still quoted today.

Grymek (1982) has drawn attention to the passage in Galen [AD 129–?199] describing the results of eating poisonous fungi when 'some have perished and some have approached death attacked by diarrhoea or "the choleric affection" or have been in danger of suffocation'. The digestive troubles are characteristic of *Amanita phalloides* poisoning while 'suffocation' (respiratory troubles), for Galen a nervous condition, could be interpreted as the effect of muscarin poisoning (see below).

Edible fungi were considered a great delicacy by the Romans and there has been some confusion between the reports of fungus poisoning and references to the use of fungi as the vehicle for the administration of poison, the most notorious instance being that of Agrippina who poisoned her husband, the emperor Claudius, on 13 October AD 54 to ensure the succession of her son Nero.

The compilers of the first printed herbals in the fifteenth and sixteenth centuries drew heavily on the classical texts and this was one factor determining the survival of some Greek and Roman views on fungi in current folklore. Concurrently it gradually became apparent that, although in the seventeenth century the first taxonomic approach to the classification of fungi was into edible and poisonous, toxicity was not a useful taxonomic criterion, that it was impossible to generalize the distinction between edible and poisonous kinds, and that the only way to distinguish the poisonous was by correct identification and to profit by the misfortunes of others.

Most fatalities in western Europe have resulted from eating *Amanita phalloides* ('death cap') and the allied *A. verna* and *A. virosa* ('destroying angel') which are extremely poisonous but in the same genus *A. muscaria* ('fly agaric') if hallucinogenic is less poisonous and *A. caesarea* ('Caesar's mushroom') and *A. rubescens* ('the blusher') are both esteemed esculents, particularly the former which was a favourite in Roman times. Other poisonous fungi are distributed through a number of genera including *Coprinus, Cortinarius, Entoloma, Galerina, Inocybe, Stropharia,* and *Tricholoma.* Some boletes (*Boletus*) are poisonous and among the larger ascomycetes *Gyromitra esculenta* ('the lorchel') may prove fatal.

There are records of fungal poisoning for many places and periods – for example the booklet by Sartory (1912) in which he summarized 61 outbreaks of poisoning in France during the summer of 1912 involving 241 victims 89 of whom died; 97 cases (51 deaths) being attributed to *Amanita phalloides* – but there are no comprehensive and reliable statistics. In the United States the National Clearing House for Poison Control Centres at Washington, DC, records *c.* 35 000 cases of accidental poisoning a year. About 1% of these are caused by eating larger fungi (*c.* 70% in children under five) but Lincoff & Mitchell (1977: 11) consider this figure to be too low. Also, concurrent interest in hallucinogenic fungi is tending to increase the incidence of mycetism as noted in the third section of this Chapter.

Toxins

The Amanita toxins proved troublesome to specify. In France J. B. L. Letellier in 1826 isolated a heat-resistant substance from a number of fungi for which he coined the name 'amanitin'. Subsequently, in collaboration with Speneux, amanitin (identified as a glucosidal alkaloid, but probably cholin)[7] and a gastro-enteric irritant were obtained from *Hypophyllum crux melitense* of Paulet, probably a variant of *Amanita phalloides.* Boudier in 1866 attributed the poisonous properties of *A. phalloides* to an alkaloid, 'bulbosine', which he failed to isolate, and in 1877 Oré named this hypothetical alkaloid 'phalloidin'. It was Kobert (1891) who first demonstrated the haemolytic properties of extracts of A. phalloides and designated the active principle 'phallin' but although the toxicity of A. phalloides was widely attributed to phallin, Kobert found that not all specimens identified as A. phalloides contained phallin and that an alcohol-soluble highly toxic substance was also present. It was the American W. W. Ford (1906) who demonstrated that A. phalloides contains a haemolysin ('amanita-haemolysis') and a heat-resistant substance ('amanita-toxin') able to induce in animals the characteristics of A. phalloides poisoning in man. The final differentiation of the A. phalloides toxins is attributable to the prolonged investigations of the Wielands, a family of German organic chemists (especially Theodor [1913–], his father and Nobel Prize winner Heinrich Otto [1877–1957], and brother Otto Heinrich [1920–]), and their colleagues (for a summary see Wieland, 1968), who proved the toxins to comprise two series of polypeptides – the amanitins ('amatoxins'; cyclic octapeptides) and the phalloidins ('phallo-toxins'; heptapeptides) – the amanitins (especially α- and β-amanitin) being many times more toxic than the phalloidins. The latter act quickly and cause gastro-intestinal symptoms, while the former act more slowly and have a strong affinity for hepatocytes and epithelial cells of the proximal convoluted tubules of the kidney.

The first fungal toxin to be isolated was muscarine (Muskarin, Germ.) from Amanita muscaria by Schmiedeberg and Koppe in 1869 and although for long mushroom poisoning in general was attributed to muscarine, this alkaloid, which is the main toxin of Inocybe patouillardii and Clitocybe dealbata, was shown to be present in very small amounts in the fly agaric. Later Schmiedeberg (1881) found another substance in A. muscaria which dilated the pupils like atropine. This he called muscaridine (the 'Pilze-atropin' of Kobert, 1906). The toxicity of the fly agaric proved to be due to isoxazole derivatives, the unstable ibotenic acid (a name derived from iboten-gu-take, Japanese for A. strobiliformis) of which muscimol is a much more highly toxic degradation product, and muscazone.

Among other toxins from larger fungi (excluding hallucinogens which are treated below) two merit mention: gyromitrin from false morels (Gyromitra spp., especially G. esculenta) and coprine present in the ink cap Coprinus atramentarius. The first was named 'helvellic acid' by Böhm & Külz (1885) and later gyromitrin when the taxa were transferred from Helvella to Gyromitra, and investigated and synthesized by List and Luft during 1967–9. At the same time studies were being made on the toxicity of monomethylhydrazine (used as a rocket propellant) at aerospace centres in the United States where the illness of workers exposed to the chemical resembled gyromitrin poisoning and it was soon established that mono-methylhydrazine is produced by the hydrolysis of gyromitrin, a reaction brought about by the acidity of the stomach.

It had been on record that drinking alcohol after eating *Coprinus atramentarius* fruit-bodies induced flushing of the face, nausea, and vomiting. Attention was drawn to the similarity of this syndrome to the Antabuse reaction – the unpleasant symptoms which follow drinking alcohol after the administration of disulfiram (Antabuse) for the treatment of chronic alcoholism – and in 1975, almost simultaneously in Sweden and the United States, the isolation from *C. atramentarius* of the compound (N^5-(1-hydroxy-cyclopropyl) L-glutamine), to which the name coprine was given (Hatfield & Shaumberg, 1975), was reported.

Prevention and treatment

Some representative examples of the prevention and treatment of mush-room poisoning in classical times have already been given. Then emesis was the most favoured treatment and the cautious Dioscorides (*Materia medica* iv, 83) offered the limiting recommendation that emetics should be eaten with the fungi. Presumably mycetism must also at times have been treated with *mithridatium*, the all-purpose antidote for poisons experimen-tally devised by King Mithridates [120–63 BC] to ensure his own immunity to poisons, and the similar *theriacs* designed to counteract the effects of venomous animals. Variants of these famous medicaments, complex formulations of up to forty or more ingredients, mostly herbal, survived in pharmacopoeias of the eighteenth and, in France and Germany, nineteenth centuries.[8]

Prevention involved offering advice on how to distinguish poisonous fungi from the edible and on diverse treatments of fungi to eliminate poisons before they came to the table. Steeping in various liquids was particularly popular. Paulet in his *Traité des Champignons* (1790–3 2: 25) stated that poisonous fungi soaked in water containing salt, vinegar, or alcohol are rendered harmless to animals and half a century later this was possibly the stimulus to his fellow countryman Frédéric Gérard, an assistant at the Jardin des Plantes in Paris, who convinced his contemporaries that soaking poisonous mushrooms in water with or without the addition of vinegar or salt and then bringing them to the boil after which they were strained

Fig. 42. Post-mark advertising the autumn exhibition of larger fungi at the Museum Nationale d'Histoire Naturelle, Paris.

off before cooking was an effective treatment. Such treatment would certainly free *Gyromitra* from gyromitrin which is water-soluble (and, it has been claimed, those cooking the fruit-bodies have been poisoned by inhalation of the toxin) but it is considered unreliable like other procedures recommended.

On the continent of Europe and in many other countries where wild edible fungi are commonly offered for sale in markets many towns and cities introduced regulations for the inspection of fungi before being marketed. In Rome, for example, inspection of all fungi offered for sale in the market was instituted in 1837.[9] Earlier in Paris, following a serious outbreak of mushroom poisoning, an ordinance was promulgated in 1754 forbidding the sale of fungi in markets and even gathering them in the environs of the city. In 1808 the sale of seven kinds of fungi was permitted and although the number was subsequently increased regulation of their sales is still in force.[10] During recent years in order to educate the public the Cryptogamic Laboratory of the Paris Museum of Natural History has each autumn organized an exhibition of larger fungi, supplemented by popular lectures (Fig. 42).

Treatments for Amanita poisoning have been many and various and although successes have been claimed no specific treatment or antidote such as the use of atropine against muscarine poisoning has yet been devised. Among the more unorthodox treatments for *Amanita phalloides* poisoning is that introduced by the Parisian doctor H. Limousin in the nineteen-thirties who fed the victim with the chopped up raw brains of seven and the stomachs of three freshly killed rabbits, the rationale underlying the treatment being that rabbits are able to eat *A. phalloides* with impunity and that there are two toxins one affecting the nervous system, the other the alimentary tract. Joseph Roques in 1821 recommended large quantities of sugared water and in 1936 Le Calvé reported success by the half-hourly administration of a teaspoonful of salt dissolved in a glass of water.

It was the bacteriologist Albert Calmette [1863–1933] of the Pasteur Institute in Paris who in 1897 first experimented with an antiserum produced in rabbits by a chloroform-water extract of *A. phalloides*. Later similar preparations were raised in sheep and finally the Pasteur Institute manufactured and distributed an antiserum prepared in horses by a method based on the investigations of Dujarric de la Rivière and others (see Dujarric de la Rivière & Heim, 1938). This antiserum was widely used and when administrated intravenously in the early stages of the poisoning was claimed to be effective.

Among other recently introduced therapeutants, thioctic acid in large doses has attracted attention and proved effective in a series of *A. phalloides* poisonings in Czechoslovakia (Kubička, 1968) and a success was also reported in the United States (Plotzker *et al.*, 1982). The Intensive Care Liver Unit at King's College Hospital, London, has successfully treated a case of Amanita poisoning by carbon-column dialysis of the patient's blood. Finally, mention may be made of the publicity recently given to the treatment devised by Dr Bastien in France which involves intravenous injection of vitamin C (ascorbic acid) supplemented by the administration of nifuroxazide and dihydrostreptomycin (Dumont *et al.*, 1981). To demonstrate his faith in this method Dr Bastien on two separate occasions ate 65–70 g of *A. phalloides*, when the treatment was successful.[11]

To simplify and accelerate the identification of toxic agarics Roy Watling and others at Edinburgh developed the on-line computerized programme as described by Margot *et al.* (1984).

2. Mycotoxicoses[12]

Like mycetism, the result of eating poisonous fungi in mistake for the edible, mycotoxicoses, the effects of ingesting toxic fungal metabolites in food frequently having no apparent connexion with fungi, has a long history; but it is only during the last twenty-five years that worldwide investigation of mycotoxicosis has become a major branch of applied mycology closely related to the even larger field of antibiotics, mycotoxins being essentially antibiotics toxic for man and higher animals, and needing the collaboration of chemists with clinicians and mycologists for their investigation.

Ergotism (ergot)

For long the only well known mycotoxicosis was ergotism usually resulting from eating rye bread prepared from flour contaminated with sclerotia of the ergot fungus (Claviceps purpurea) which replace the ovaries of the rye (and also other cereals and grasses) (Fig. 43). In recent times ergot has been best known as a drug used at childbirth, formerly to hasten labour but now almost exclusively post partem to reduce the risk of post-partem haemorrhage. Its status as a drug has followed that of other natural products as noted in Chapter 6. At first officially recognized by the British Pharmacopoeia, it was subsequently relegated to the British Pharmaceutical Codex where in the current 1979 edition it has been replaced by the active ingredients ergometrine maleate and ergometrine tartrate. While the use of ergot as a drug extends back to ancient times, ergotism, the effects on man of eating ergot-contaminated food, has an equally long history which has been well documented by a number of authors[13] – including George Barger [1878–1939], the British chemist who made pioneering studies on the ergot alkaloids, summarized in his Ergot and Ergotism, 1931, based on the Dohme lectures delivered in 1928 at Johns Hopkins University, Baltimore – who may be consulted to supplement the present outline.

The first unambiguous published reference to ergot is that by the herbalist Adam Lonitzer (Lonicerus) in his Kreuterbuch of 1582 and ergot was first illustrated in Gaspar Bauhin's Theatri botanici, 1658, where, following his brother Jean Bauhin, ergoted rye is treated as a distinct species 'Secale luxurians'. It was not until 1853 that the French lawyer Louis-René Tulasne elucidated the life history of the ergot fungus and proposed the new genus Claviceps to accommodate it (Fig. 43).[14]

The use of ergot was, however, known to the Chinese (Chou King [1100 BC] mentions ergot as an obstetrical remedy[15]) and it has been suggested that the numerous recommendations by Hippocrates to use barley flour cooked and mixed with water as a drink to further childbirth and in formulations for other uterine complaints were because the barley was ergotized. Dioscorides' recommendation of wheat flour cooked with water for haemoptysis (bleeding from the lungs) is a parallel case where ergotization of the wheat might have ensured success.[16] There has also been speculation among classical scholars of the meaning of the Greek word 'melanthium' which is constantly associated with remedies for disorders of the uterus. It has most frequently been interpreted as the name of plants of the genus Nigella (family Ranunculacae) but occasionally the word has been translated as ergot.[17] The Persian physician Abu Mansur

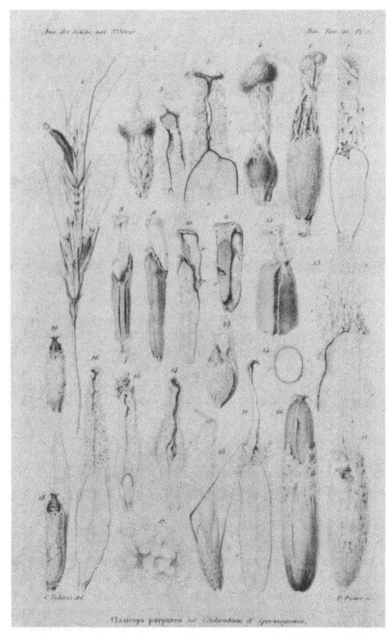

Fig. 43. Sclerotia of ergot (*Claviceps purpurea*). (Tulasne, 1853, plate i.)

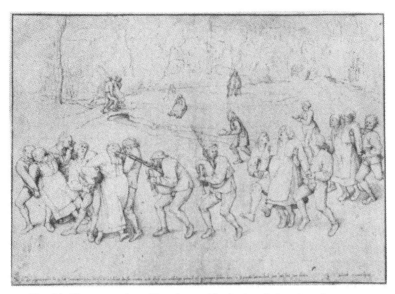

Fig. 44. Choreomaniacs. Dancing at Moelenbeeck Sint Jans [now part of Brussels] on St John's Day, 1564 by Pieter Brugel the Elder [1528–69]. Each of the afflicted women, who show signs consistent with convulsive ergotism, is supported by two men. Crossing water was an essential feature of the dance; bagpipes the traditional accompaniment.

Muwaffak bino Ali Harawi mentioned ergot in the 10th century AD but it is with the medieval references to what is now known as ergotism that firmer ground is reached.

Two main types of ergot poisoning of man were differentiated as the gangrenous or necrotic ('morbus necroticus') and the convulsive. The first, which in Europe most often occurred in France and countries west of the Rhine, is initiated by intense burning sensations and irritation in the limbs, which slowly mortify and may spontaneously drop off while the second, which has been associated, but doubtfully, with vitamin A deficiency, and was most frequently recorded from Germany and Russia, results in spasms, convulsions, and rigidity (which may be confused with epilepsy), and a ravenous hunger. From the Middle Ages up to the end of the nineteenth century outbreaks of ergotism of epidemic proportions were regularly reported from most European countries (the first from France in AD 857)[18], generally following wet cold summers and starvation conditions in winter. Professor Backman (1952) has assembled convincing evidence for attributing dancing epidemics of medieval times to convulsive ergotism

(Fig. 44), the effects of which were attributed to possession by the devil. Appeals were made to various saints including St Généviève [422–502] (the patron saint of Paris), St Vitonus, and especially St Antony the Hermit [b. 251] who because he resisted the temptations to which he was exposed in the Egyptian desert became the most important demon-expeller of the Catholic saints and was by tradition in charge of the flames through which all who entered the heavenly Paradise had to pass and which the saint could intensify or reduce. Thus ergotism, or *ignus sacer* [holy fire][19] as it was called, became known as St Antony's Fire and in 1095 Pope Urban II founded the order of St Antony to take care of those afflicted by the Fire.

From the end of the sixteenth century dancing epidemics ceased. Sufferers no longer attributed the 'dance' to the devil but to some sort of impurity in the grain and those affected were said to have *Die Kriebelkrankheit*. In 1597 the Medical Faculty at Marburg decided that a local outbreak was caused by yarrow (*Achilea*), mixed with the grain. Thuillier *père* in 1630 attributed *ignis sacer* to corn smut and undertook feeding experiments on hens with toxic rye which induced the characteristic changes in the comb. Subsequently, Denis Dodart [1634–1737] a Parisian lawyer with botanical leanings and physician to Louis XIV, in 1676 wrote a long letter to the Acadème Royale des Sciences on an epidemic of ergotism that had recently occurred in areas south of Paris which he associated with the consumption of degenerated rye, characterized by black grains white within. He observed that the severity of the disease was directly related to the amount of degenerated rye consumed and noted that it exerted its greatest influence when fresh when it led to blocked milk flow in nursing mothers, fever, and scurvy-like effects. He recommended that the authorities compelled the rye to be sieved to remove the ergot before use. A century later Carl Linnaeus thought that admixture of the rye with radish (*Raphanus*) caused ergotism which he designated Raphania.[20]

Ergotism is no longer a medical problem (the last notable outbreak in England was in 1927 among a small rye-bread-eating community in Manchester; Robertson & Ashly, 1928; Morgan 1929) and a relatively minor one for veterinarians. In cattle and other farm animals the usual symptoms of ergotism are the gangrenous and although abortion has been frequently said to be an expression of ergotism there is little convincing evidence to support the claim.[21] Although rye has been the usual source of ergotism in man *C. purpurea* and its many intraspecific variants attack a wide range of grasses attractive to cattle and as the sclerotia only develop on grass at its maturity measures to prevent the grass seeding have given some measure of control.

Ergotism of grasses of the genus *Paspalum* is caused by a different species, *C. paspali*, and ergotism induced in cattle, sheep, and horses grazing infected grass has since 1916 been distinguished as 'paspalum staggers' of which the symptoms are largely nervous. Cattle and equines develop a trembling of the muscles and if moved definite ataxia, and when frightened uncoordinated movement results in their falling over in curious attitudes (Hopkirk, 1936). Paspalum staggers has been reported from North America, Africa, Australia and New Zealand, Europe (Portugal), and Russia (Sarkisov, 1954).

During recent years much research was directed towards identifying the cause of 'rye-grass staggers' of New Zealand and sporadically reported elsewhere the symptoms of which show similarities to paspalum staggers. Ergotization was ruled out and the incrimination of penicillia inconclusive. In 1981, Fletcher and Harvey offered compelling evidence that the toxicity of the rye-grass is due to the slow-growing fungal endophyte which occurs as a layer of mycelium in some seeds of *Lolium temulentum* and *L. perenne* as described by Kathleen Sampson and others[22] more than fifty years ago. Concurrently, Gallagher and his colleagues chemically defined two of the active principles as new mycotoxins, lolitrem A and B.

Russian and Japanese investigations

It was in Russia and Japan that germinal work on mycotoxicoses was undertaken. In Russia, in addition to ergotism and paspalum staggers, a series of mycotoxicoses associated with mouldy cereals and fodder have attracted attention for more than a century. During the eighteen-sixties Kashin-Beck (or Urov) disease (a disease of childhood characterized by a 'chronic disabling, degenerative, generalized osteoarthritis') was prevalent among the Cossacks and later established as endemic in both Asiatic and European Russia and the northern parts of China and Korea. Incidence of the disorder was said to have been reduced by importing wholesome grain into the affected areas. The same, or a very similar mycotoxicosis characterized by the 'drunken (or intoxicating) bread syndrome' was, in 1916, the subject of a book by the famous Russian mycologist and plant pathologist N. A. Naumov [1888–1959] who identified the causal fungi as *Giberella saubinetii* [*G. zeae*] and *Fusarium subulatum*. Eating bread made from infected cereals caused headache, general weakness, nausea, and vomiting.

A now well established mycotoxicosis is *alimentary toxic aleukia* (ATA) or septic angina, a widespread haemorrhagic disease in Russia. Known before the First World War, it attained epidemic proportions during the Second,

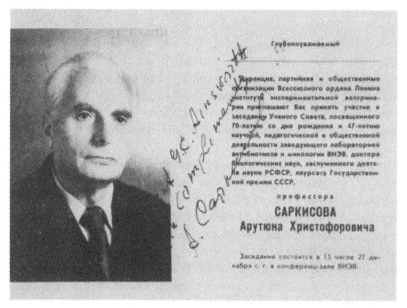

Fig. 45. A. K. Sarkisov, aet. 70.

especially in the Orenburg district where in 1944 more than 10% of the
population was affected and a special regional laboratory was established
to study all aspects of ATA. In the affected districts it was common practice
to allow the ripe cereals (wheat, barley, rye, oats, prosomillet (*Panicum*
supp.), and buckwheat (*Fagopyrum esculentum*)) to overwinter under the
snow cover and to postpone harvesting until spring. This encouraged
fungal infection of the grain, especially when the snow cover was
exceptionally deep so that the underlying soil did not freeze to its usual
depth, and when the spring was warm resulting in frequent thawing and
freezing. The symptoms which appear two to three weeks after eating toxic
grain, include a haemorrhagic skin rash, bleeding from the nose and
throat, exhaustion of the bone marrow and death may occur a month or
so later. The toxin responsible was first experimentally shown to be
produced by *Fusarium sporotrichoides* and *F. poae* but later a number of
other fungi isolated from overwintered grain were found to produce
toxins, those mainly responsible for ATA being trichothecenes, the toxicity
of which could be assessed by a skin test on rabbits. A large literature was
generated.[23]

In the early nineteen-thirties *stachybotryotoxicosis* (Fig. 46) caused the
death of thousands of horses in the Ukraine during the winter months,

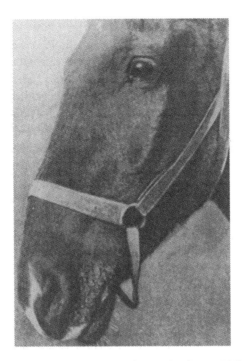

Fig. 46. Stachybotryotoxicosis in a horse. (Sarkisov, 1954, fig. 61).

when the animals are stabled, and intensive work undertaken during the next decade and since showed the cause to be a mycotoxin (satrotoxin (stachybotryotoxin); a series of trichothecens) resulting from infection of the straw by *Stachybotrys alternans* [*S. atra*]. Cattle, man, and animals in zoological gardens were also shown to be susceptible.[24]

In Japan, cardiac beriberi (Shoshin-Kakke)[25], characterized by paralysis, cardiovascular damage, and respiratory failure resulting in death within three days was known in the seventeenth century. In 1891 Sakaki recognized the connexion of the disorder with eating mouldy rice and demonstrated the toxicity of the mouldy rice to rabbits, guinea pigs, and frogs. From the introduction in 1910 of rice inspection to prevent the marketing of damaged grain the incidence of cardiac beriberi declined but it was not until 1940 that I. Miyake *et al.* isolated the toxin-producing mould which they thought to be undescribed so they named it *Penicillium toxicarium*, later shown to be a synonym of *P. citreo-viride* Biourge. Subsequently Hirata (1947) isolated the toxin, *citreoviridin*, a nonaketide.

After the Second World War some of the rice which had to be imported into Japan had deteriorated in store and a second mycotoxicosis associated with 'yellowed rice' occurred. Among the fungi isolated from the defective rice were *Penicillium citreo-viride, P. citrinum,* and *P. islandicum* (all rich in anthraquinones), the last yielding a series of related toxins including *islandicin* (islanditoxin), *cyclochlorotine, leuteoskyrin,* and *rugulosin,* able to induce liver damage (cirrhosis; and the first two hepatoma).[26]

These investigations were largely ignored outside Russia and Japan, in part due to language difficulties (few microbiologists in the west having first-hand access to literature written in Russian or Japanese), in part to the relative isolation of Russian investigators, and in part to the lack of appreciation shown by both the veterinary and medical professions of the potentialities of fungi. There were a few notable exceptions. As early as 1933 D. G. Steyn, Veterinary Research Officer at Onderspoort, South Africa, concluded after a comprehensive review of published records and his own feeding experiments on rabbits that 'For all practical purposes fungus-infected foodstuffs must be considered poisonous until the contrary has been proved by extensive feeding experiments in the different classes of stock'. Twenty years later the investigations by Forgacs and Caarl in the United States and their propaganda on behalf of mycotoxicoses did much to keep the topic alive. A complete change of attitude occurred within a few years largely as the result of the elucidation of two rather spectacular mycotoxicoses: facial eczema of sheep and cattle in New Zealand and aflatoxicosis of poultry in the United Kingdom.

Facial eczema or pithomycotoxicosis (sporidesmin)[27]

Facial eczema of sheep and cattle, a hepatitis accompanied by jaundice and by photosensitization of non- or lightly pigmented skin surfaces, was observed in New Zealand as long ago as 1898 (and Charles Darwin noted a rather similar disorder of horses in England in 1868[28]) but it attracted little attention before a disastrous outbreak in 1938 when several million sheep and many diary herds were affected throughout the North Island since when there have been sporadic economically important outbreaks. Failure to transmit the disease from affected to healthy animals led to the disorder being attributed to 'dietetic errors'. The correlation of the incidence of facial eczema with rapidly growing pastures following warm autumn rains suggested that the toxic material was present in such pastures but experimental feeding trials were hampered by the affected pastures rapidly becoming 'safe' and the first successful induction of the disease by experimental feeding was not until 1941. Although the toxin was not isolated chemical investigation of toxic feed led to the development of a chemical test, the so-called 'beaker test', for the toxic principle which at first was taken to be a toxin produced by the grass, no evidence having been obtained to implicate any of some 1 600 micro-organisms isolated from affected pastures. Pastures were sampled by mowing and in 1958 a breakthrough occurred when the scrapings from a gang mower which gave a positive 'beaker test' were found to be composed mainly of fungal spores. Cultures yielded spores which when fed to guinea-pigs and sheep were found to induce the typical facial eczema syndrome (Percival & Thornton, 1958). Identification of the fungus caused some confusion. It was at first designated *Sporidesmium bakeri* (Thornton & Percival, 1959) (hence the name *sporidesmin* for the toxic principle, a series of piperazine derivatives) but M. B. Ellis of the Commonwealth Mycological Institute later showed this binomial to be a synonym of *Pithomyces chartarum*.[29]

Facial eczema has also been recorded in Australia (Victoria)[30] and South Africa and air-borne spores of *P. chartarum* have been detected in Great Britain[31] where facial eczema has not been observed.

Aflatoxicosis (aflatoxin)

Sir, – Since the end of May we have encountered 45 outbreaks of 'disease' in turkey poults associated with high mortality and constant *post-mortem* lesions. Birds died in good condition after a very short illness and mortality rates ranged from 10 to 70 per cent. Affected birds were usually about 4 weeks old, but birds 12 to 15 weeks old were sometimes involved.

These opening words of a letter to *The Veterinary Record* of 30 July 1960 from a group of workers at the Veterinary Investigation Centre and the School of Veterinary Medicine, Cambridge (see Stevens *et al.*, 1960) initiated a major branch of applied mycological research which still flourishes a quarter of a century later. It has been estimated that during the summer of 1960 more than 100000 young turkeys,[32] 14000 ducklings,[33] and also many young pheasants and partridges in the United Kingdom died after being fed rations containing groundnut (or peanut, *Arachis hypogea*) meal. Concurrently outbreaks of disease associated with feeding the same importation of Brazilian groundnut meal were reported in cattle,[34] pigs,[35] and, experimentally, in sheep. In all these animals acute liver damage was a prominent feature. Added interest was aroused by the finding that rats fed on a diet of toxic groundnut meal showed no immediate response but after six months developed cancer of the liver[36] and cows fed on hay and a concentrate ration containing 20% toxic groundnut meal secreted the toxin in the milk.[37] There was much speculation regarding the cause of what came to be known as 'turkey X disease' and the stages by which the problem was solved as summarized by P. K. C. Austwick[38] provide an interesting example of the lack of awareness of the potentiality of fungi as toxin producers prevalent in the country at the time.

Because of the heavy losses among poultry already referred to the Agricultural Research Council in August 1960 convened a meeting of representatives of all branches of the poultry industry together with veterinarians and others at which there was a general consensus that a toxin was present in the feed.[39] The effects of the toxin resembled those of *Senecio* (ragwort) poisoning and in the September Austwick, then mycologist at the Central Veterinary Laboratory, Weybridge, was asked to make a comparative examination of a toxic sample of Brazilian groundnut meal, which the veterinarian W. P. Blount[40] had suggested was the suspicious ingredient, and a non-toxic sample of Indian origin. No evidence of toxic plant material was found but microscopic examination showed fungal hyphae in approximately 20% of the groundnut cotyledon fragments of the toxic, but not the non-toxic, sample and Dr Mary Noble, seed pathologist of the Department of Agriculture for Scotland, Edinburgh, confirmed that the cotyledons appeared to have been invaded around harvest time. This was the first evidence for the possible implication of fungi. Most of the affected groundnut fragments were easily distinguished by their darker colour but culture proved negative, the mycelium presumably being dead. In spite of these findings the idea that the toxicity had a mycotic origin found little support and up to June 1961 only six additional meal samples had been examined, hyphae being detected in five toxic samples but not in one non-toxic. Blount, chief scientific adviser to the British Oil and Cake Mills which had imported 5000 tons of Brazilian groundnut meal early in 1960 and incorporated it in feed at 2.5 to 18% as a source of protein, in the autumn of 1960 visited Brazil where he learnt that there had been problems with crops from wet harvesting seasons but he did not associate this with the likelihood that wet seasons provided suitable conditions for fungal growth in the newly harvested crop. It was in July 1961 that the director of the Central Veterinary Laboratory asked Austwick to assist 'in an advisory capacity' the Tropical Products Institute, London, where the toxin was being studied, on the possibility that the groundnut poison was of mycotic origin and arrangements were made for attempts at isolating toxin-producing fungi from an extremely mouldy sample of Ugandan groundnuts which had caused outbreaks of toxicosis of ducklings in Kenya. At both laboratories a toxin-producing mould was isolated and identified by J. J. Elphick of the Commonwealth Mycological Institute, Kew, as *Aspergillus parasiticus* (a member of the *Aspergillus flavus-oryzae* group) the type culture of which was found to produce a similar toxin. Letters on the carcinogenic effect on rats, as determined at the Unilever Research Laboratory, Sharnbrook, and on the mycotic origin of the toxicity were submitted to *Nature* and announced for simultaneous publication in September 1961 but at the last moment the letters were withdrawn, because, as the scientific correspondent of a national newspaper discovered, of a complaint about the specific mention of Canadian maize as an additional source of the toxin. Amended letters appeared in the December (Lancaster *et al.*, 1961; Sargeant, Sheridan *et al.*, 1961) and caused a considerable stir in groundnut-producing countries which, fearing loss of exports, made representations to the British Government which took the unprecedented step of placing an embargo on further publication of research articles on the topic by workers at the two laboratories chiefly concerned. This embargo lasted until the mimeographed report of an Interdepartmental Working Party on Groundnut Toxicity Research was circulated in June 1962 (and officially released on 15 August). It was in this report that the name *aflatoxin* (*A. flavus* toxin) was coined and one of the conclusions reached was that the hazards to human health in the United Kingdom from aflatoxin were minimal. A different attitude was taken by commercial concerns and a groundnut-containing baby food designed as a protein supplement to combat malnutrition was withdrawn from the market. Subsequent food analyses showed aflatoxin to be of widespread occurrence in both animal and human food and in several parts of Africa and Southeast Asia ingestion of aflatoxins has been correlated with the incidence of chronic liver disease.

Aflatoxin was also shown to cause hepatoma in trout (*Salmo*) fed with pellets of meat, fish, and vegetable meals (Ashley *et al.*, 1965; Sinnhuber *et al.*, 1965).[41]

At first the assay of aflatoxin was by biological testing in 1-day-old ducklings (Sargeant, O'Kelley *et al.*, 1961), to which 20 μg aflatoxin is fatal in 24 h, and a fluorescence test was developed for detecting its presence. Further chemical work showed aflatoxin to have two components, B and C, the former subsequently being divided into aflatoxin B_1 and B_2. This work culminated in the chemical characterization of the group as a series of bisfuranocoumarin compounds and the synthesis of aflatoxin B_1, a powerful carcinogen.

If aflatoxin was proposed as a food additive, it would be banned, but because of the harvesting practices in producing countries where the standard of agricultural practice is often low and of the conditions of high temperature and humidity under which harvested groundnuts are stored the elimination of the moulding of groundnuts is a long-term project. A legal requirement for the absence of aflatoxin in groundnuts would therefore be detrimental to the economy of the producing countries and so in 1964 the United States Food & Drug Administration established an aflatoxin tolerance of 20 ppb for peanuts, later adjusted to 25 ppb for raw peanuts and 20 ppb for finished products containing peanuts, and also for animal feed ingredients.[42]

Although the outbreak of 'turkey X disease' in the United Kingdom was an isolated incident, as Austwick concluded:

The effect of this episode in avian disease was to initiate a new research industry which removed mycotoxins from their regional obscurity and presented them as disease-producing agents whose exploitation as experimental research tools has enabled important advances to be made in our understanding of the biological mechanisms of toxicity and carcinogenicity.[43]

Today, twenty-five years after its discovery, study of aflatoxin still flourishes.[44] There have been two major monographs[45] on the aflatoxins, dozens of reviews,[46] and hundreds of papers reporting the results of research which may be consulted for further details.

Some representative mycotoxins

The explosion of interest, especially in the United States, in mycotoxins and particularly aflatoxin was mainly due to the carcinogenic effect of the latter. Many economically significant mycotoxicoses of animals were defined but fewer among humans because of the difficulties of experimenting on man for whom evidence for the involvement of mycotoxins is mainly statistical. As with the macrofungi, attempts to correlate toxin production by microfungi with the taxonomy or ecology of the toxin-producing species yields no distinctive pattern.

Other important mycotoxins which have attracted attention include:

Citrinin (a pentaketide) produced by *Penicillium citrinum* and other Penicillium species was first described by A. C. Hetherington and Raistrick in 1931 and recognized as an antibacterial antibiotic ten years later by Raistrick & G. Smith (1941). Krogh *et al.*, (1970) showed citrinin to be a cause of nephropathy of pigs in Denmark.

Dicoumarol toxin (3,3-methylene*bis*(4-hydrocoumarin)) produced by strains of *Aspergillus*, *Penicillium*, and *Mucor* infecting sweet clover (*Melilotus*) causes symptoms resembling haemorrhagic septicaemia in cattle, horses, and sheep. It was first recorded from the United States (Paulman, 1923) and shortly afterwards from Canada (Schofield, 1924).[47]

Ochratoxin A (another coumarin derivative; Van der Merwe *et al.*, 1965) produced by *Penicillium viridicatum* and other penicillia causes mycotic nephropathy in pigs which has been much investigated by Palle Krogh and others in Denmark where it was first described in 1928.[48]

Patulin (clavicin, claviformin, expansin, penicidin; a tetraketide), a metabolite of *Penicillium patulum* and many other penicillia and aspergilli. Like citrinin, it was first known as an antibiotic. In 1954 T. Yamamoto[49] and others attributed the death of more than a hundred dairy cows in Japan to a patulin-containing dry malt feed.

Rubratoxin A and *B* (nonadrides), produced by *Penicillium rubrum, P. purpurogenum,* and *Aspergillus flavus,* have caused hepatitis in cattle and pigs in the United States (Burnside *et al.*, 1957).

Zearalenone (or F2) (a phenolic macrolide) produced by *Fusarium* spp., including *F. graminearum* (anamorph of *Giberella zeae*) and the cause of vulvovaginitis in pigs worldwide was first reported from the United States by Buxton (1926). R. McKay (professor of Plant Pathology, Dublin) was the first to isolate *F. graminearum* from toxic barley (see McErlean, 1952).

Finally, mention may be made of two mycotoxicoses, in which plant-pathogenic fungi are involved, with unusual clinical features: the salivary syndrome in cattle and horses and photodermatitis of workers handling celery (*Apium graveolens*). The first, recognized by farmers in the Midwest of the United States for more than thirty years, is characterized by excessive salivation of animals fed red clover (*Trifolium pratense*) hay (O'Dell *et al.*, 1959) and Smalley *et al.* (1962) showed the toxicity to be associated with infection of the clover by *Rhizoctonia leguminicola* which when grown in pure culture was found to yield a toxic metabolite, *slaframine* (1 S,6 S,8a S)-l-acetoxy-6-amino-octahydroindolizine),[50] able to induce a similar response *in vivo.*

The second, first recorded in France in 1926 and attributed to celery oil, was first experimentally associated with celery attacked by pink rot caused by *Sclerotia sclerotiorum* by Birmingham *et al.* (1961) in the United States and in 1963 Scheel *et al.* characterized two phototoxic furanocoumarin metabolites (psoralens) from diseased celery as *xanthotoxin* and 4,5′,8-trimethylpsoralen.

3. Hallucinogenic fungi

During recent years there has been much interest in hallucinogenic fungi. Since time immemorial man has employed intoxicants. Every region has its range of alcoholic beverages derived by fungal and bacterial fermentation and many plant products have been valued for their intoxicating properties. Until the nineteen-fifties the only well known mycological example was the use of the fruit-bodies of *Muchumor* (the fly agaric, *Amanita muscaria*) by certain north-eastern Siberian tribes, particularly the Chukchi, Koryak, and Kamchadal of Kamchatka, as recorded by explorers and travellers since the seventeenth century.[51] Dry fruit-bodies, which are much valued and exchanged with the tribesmen by Russian traders for furs, are stored for use on special occasions when after being soaked in water or chewed they are swallowed to induce intoxication, hallucinations, and uncontrolled excited dancing. The active principle is excreted in the urine which is collected and drunk to prolong the intoxication. Much interest was aroused by Wasson's study from which he concluded that the Soma of the Indian Rig Veda, which was at the same time 'a god, a plant, and the juice of that plant' and on the identity of which there had been much speculation, should be equated with the fly agaric (Wasson, 1968) while concurrently the Semitic philologist John Allegro in *The sacred mushroom and the cross*, 1970, implicated the fly agaric with cults underlying Christianity.

Two poetical references to hallucinogens are not without interest. Coleridge in the closing lines of Kubla Khan – the only fragment he could recollect of a longer poem which came to him during drug-induced sleep – indicated the high state – 'His flashing eyes, his floating hair!' – of him who:

'...on honey-dew hath fed
And drunk the milk of Paradise',

while few of those who sing Whittier's famous hymn 'Dear Lord and Father of mankind' realize that the 'foolish ways' for which they ask forgiveness is the use of 'heathen soma' still, metaphorically, brewed 'in many a Christian fane', and to which the first ten verses of the poem, entitled 'The brewing of soma', from which the hymn is taken, are devoted. Whether Coleridge's 'honey-dew' had any connexion with the honey-dew of the ergot fungus, which contains lysergic acid derivatives, must remain obscure and no clue has been found to Whittier's interest in soma.

The use of hallucinogenic fungi is a practice of long standing in parts of Central America. In Guatemala the highland Maya carved 'mushroom stones' of uncertain significance which have been dated around the beginning of the present millennium and fungi are featured in the three Maya codices to have survived.[52] When Cortez conquered the adjacent Mexico in the sixteenth century the Aztecs were found to be using mushrooms (teonanácatl, God's flesh) in their religious rites and such practices have survived to the present day but overlaid with Christian symbolism acquired from the Spanish missionary friars. During this century use of hallucinogenic fungi was confused with that of the peyote cactus (Lophophora williamsii) and apparently it was the Mexican botanist Blas Pablo Reko who, in 1919, first established the survival of teonanácatl, an observation subsequently confirmed by the anthropologist Roberto J. Weitlauder[53] and the ethnobotanist Richard Schultes.[53] The main thrust in the modern interest in hallucinogenic fungi originated from the ethnomycological studies of the New York banker R. Gordon Wasson and his medically trained Russian-born wife Valentina P. Wasson [1901–58]. The former at the time of their wedding in 1926 was a mycophobe, the latter a mycophile, and it was to seek an explanation of this cultural cleavage that the Wassons initiated their scholarly and wide-ranging research.

It was on the night of 29–30 June 1955 that Wasson and Allan Richardson (a New York society photographer) in a remote Mexican village attended their first mushroom ceremony led by two women, mother and daughter, who were both Mexeteco-speaking curanderas, or shamans, and at first hand verified the powerful hallucinogenic properties of the fungi employed.[54] Subsequently, with the help of Roger Heim of the Paris Natural History Museum the fungi were described, identified as representatives of several genera (especially Psilocybe, several new species of which were proposed), and handsomely monographed (Heim et al., 1958, 1967; Singer & Smith, 1958). Psilocybe mexicana and other species were cultured (first at the Paris Museum) and two psychotropic active principles, psilocybin and psilocin, chemically defined and synthesized by Albert Hofmann and his colleagues at the Sandoz laboratories, Basel.

Attention to hallucinogenic fungi was reinforced and popularized by the writings of Aldous Huxley, R. D. Laing, and other authors and their self-experimentation to induce psychotropic effects, with mescaline (the active alkaloid of the peyote cactus) and LSD (lysergic acid diethylamide). It was also found that certain widely distributed species of *Psilocybe* (such as the 'liberty cap' (*P. semilanceata*), common on grassland) were hallucinogenic and these were much collected both for personal use and for sale. As a result increasing numbers of the participants have had to receive medical treatment.[55] Psilocin in England became a class A drug but the legislation is somewhat anomalous for though the possession of psilocin and the sale of psilocin-containing agaric fruit-bodies is illegal it is not an offence to have possession of naturally occurring material which incidentally contains a controlled drug, cannabis plants being an exception.

9

Training mycopathologists: an educational problem[1]

Before considering the formal training of a mycopathologist, attention must be drawn to aspects of the training of a mycologist which is, in general, a twentieth century innovation. Early mycologists were mostly self-taught or had developed an interest and knowledge of fungi by their association with others of similar inclination. The most frequent professional qualifications of the first mycologists were medicine and the church. As in other branches of natural history mycology was for long dominated by amateurs but during recent years they have lost much ground to professionals – even in the study of toadstools. For example, during the first half of the life of the British Mycological Society – 90 years old in 1986 – the President was an amateur on 16 occasions, during the second half only twice and the last time was 30 years ago.

It has never been particularly easy to obtain a formal training in mycology. Botany and zoology have for long received university recognition and fungi being traditionally considered plants (if only on the basis that they were not animals) have been treated as part of botany. Whether mycology received special attention depended (and still depends) largely on the interests of the reigning professor. Only two English universities – Cambridge and the Imperial College of Science & Technology (a school of London University) – have maintained a long-term interest in mycology and at both these centres there has been a strong plant-pathological bias. Mycology has not fared much better as a branch of microbiology in which many universities have invested. In spite of this there is today throughout the world more interest in mycology in universities and technical institutes than ever before and this interest is at a higher level.

As already inferred, the traditional entry into mycology is via a first degree in botany, a mycological interest having developed during undergraduate studies. This is an advantage for a career in phytopathology but not nearly so useful for one in mycopathology. Should a student be sufficiently eccentric to enter a university with the idea of becoming a mycopathologist already in mind then a first degree in microbiology biased towards mycology is probably the most helpful. The next stage in a mycological career is normally to work on some mycological topic for a higher degree and that is still the best method. The particular mycological topic does not greatly matter. To gain the maximum mycological experience is clearly the only guide for the potential mycopathologist for the calls on his expertise are now so wide. They range over the classical pathogenic fungi, 'opportunistic' pathogens, and the larger poisonous fungi to those causing mycotoxicoses or associated with allergic conditions. Much of the recent pre-eminence in mycopathology in North America has been associated with mycopathologists who were sound mycologists. For instance, Chester Emmons' first research was on *Penicillium*, Ajello's on chytrids – and both did postgraduate work under outstanding mycologists before they entered the mycopathological field.

The university is not however, the only route into mycopathology for a non-medical. The skills required by laboratory technicians both widen and deepen and in large diagnostic laboratories there are clear openings for specialization in the identification and manipulation of fungi. Aspects of mycological knowledge and skills are, indeed, a requirement for professional qualifications in medical laboratory technology and a number of useful contributions have already been made to mycopathology by workers in this field.

Of the initial training of the clinician – whether medical or veterinary – little need be said. It seems that with the undergraduate courses in both these disciplines so overloaded the amount of mycological instruction will be minimal and it may still be a not-unreasonable suspicion that apart from ringworm and thrush the average medical or veterinary undergraduate hears little about mycoses. But again, as for mycology, the position is on the whole better than it ever has been.

Recruits to mycopathology are thus drawn from clinicians who may know little about fungi and their ecology, mycologists or microbiologists who know more about fungi in general but are unfamiliar with the common pathogenic species and with methods of medical diagnosis, and laboratory technicians familiar with varied pathological material and a few fungi which need to be set in broader perspective. Finally there are a few biochemists and serologists who need to acquire some knowledge of fungi and mycoses. How have these needs been met?

Medical and veterinary mycological teaching may be considered to have originated in France during the last decade of the nineteenth century and the first quarter of the twentieth when the subject was dominated by Sabouraud and his French contemporaries including Blanchard, de

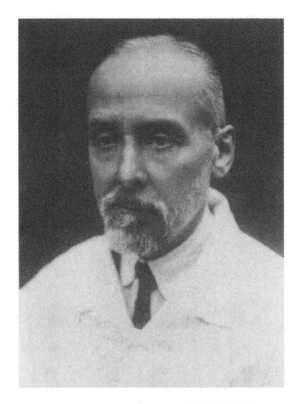

Fig. 47. Maurice Langeron (1874–1950).

Beurmann, and Gougerot in Paris and Bodin in Rennes. Sabouraud never did much formal mycological teaching although the St Louis Hospital in Paris where he worked became a centre for pilgrimage by dermatologists from all parts of the world. Mycoses of animals and man were one of the parasitologist Nevue-Lemaire's interests both before and after the First World War and in the twenties the bacteriologist Auguste Sartory of the University of Nancy wrote several textbooks on medical mycology based on his own lectures. In the inter-war years it was Maurice Langeron (Fig. 47) of the Faculty of Medicine of the University of Paris who regularly offered courses in medical mycology of the grade Certificat D'Études Spéciales (CES) and among his students who distinguished themselves in medical mycology were M. Ota, S. Milochevitch, R. V. Talice, P. Guerra, M. Baeza, and R. Vanbreuseghem. Concurrently, Castellani gave sporadic courses of lectures in England (and the United States) where little development occurred until J. T. Duncan (Fig. 48) (see Chapter 10), after

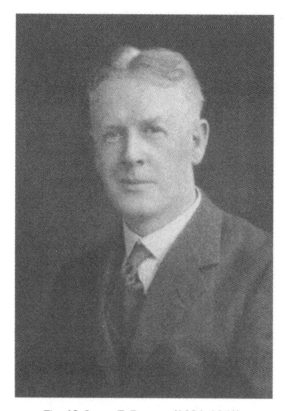

Fig. 48. James T. Duncan (1884–1958).

service as pathologist in Singapore, took up a post as bacteriologist at the London School of Hygiene & Tropical Medicine and developed a deep interest in fungi. At first he lectured to the Diploma of Bacteriology class on industrial mycology and when this topic was taken over by George Smith he continued to instruct the same class on medical mycology until his retirement in 1949 by which time he had been appointed the first Reader in Medical Mycology in London University. Duncan was a stimulating teacher. His lectures were wide ranging and the accompanying demonstrations meticulously prepared. He was extremely knowledgeable and the true measure of his stature is given by the large number of papers published by others in which acknowledgement is made to Duncan for help, guidance, or inspiration. Unfortunately Duncan was a perfectionist. He had difficulty in bringing anything to a conclusion and a large and comprehensive manuscript for a textbook, constantly under revision, was never completed. Much of his wide experience was thus lost to us.

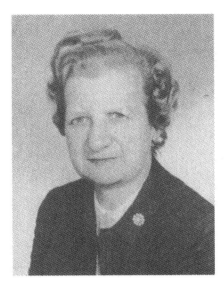

Fig. 49. Rhoda W. Benham (1894–1957).

The inspiration for many of the current postgraduate courses in mycopathology originated in North America. In the United States courses in microbiology started about 1870 at Harvard University where the mycologist Carol W. Dodge offered his first course in medical mycology in 1924 to two dermatologists. Arthur T. Henrici in his bacteriological course at the University of Minnesota, Minneapolis, on the evidence of his 1930 textbook, presumably introduced some medical mycology while a year or two earlier Joseph Gardner Hopkins, head of the Dermatology Department in the College of Physicians and Surgeons, New York (which is the medical school of Columbia University) appointed Rhoda W. Benham (Fig. 49), a botany graduate of Barnard College, to work in the diagnostic laboratory of his Department where she gained a doctorate for a taxonomic and serological study in *Candida*. In collaboration with Professor Hopkins and Bernard O. Dodge (cousin of C. W. Dodge), mycologist and plant pathologist at the New York Botanical Garden, Rhoda Benham organized a comprehensive postgraduate course on medical mycology. Among the many who worked or studied in her laboratory (the first of its kind in the United States) were Chester Emmons, Mary E. Hopper, Arturo L. Carrión, Lucille Georg, and Margarita Silva.

The most famous North American course in medical mycology is the annual summer course offered at Duke University. This was started in 1947 by Norman Conant (Fig. 50) and his colleagues and after Professor

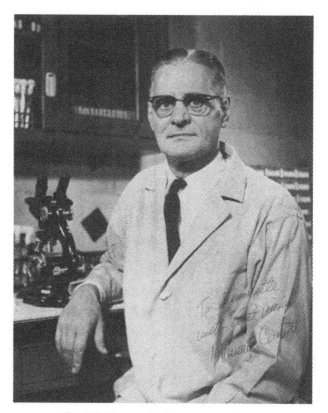

Fig. 50. Norman F. Conant (1908–84).

Conant's retirement has been continued by Dr T. Mitchell. The course has been attended by workers from all parts of the world. It is open to clinicians, pathologists, bacteriologists, mycologists, and technicians, and runs for a month with classes on six days a week. Lectures, practical work, and demonstrations are given by members of the departments of medicine, pathology, and bacteriology and there is emphasis on the clinical, pathological, and therapeutic aspects of fungal infections. Patients, clinical materials, cultures, and laboratory animals are available for study, according to the prospectus, while practical laboratory aids which help to establish a definite diagnosis are stressed. The course concludes with an examination.

A number of similar courses are now available in the United States. The annual list of summer courses listed each year by the Mycological Society of America usually includes several of mycopathological interest.

Another very useful training project, originated by Ajello at Atlanta,

Georgia, in collaboration with the Audio-Visual Section (then based at Atlanta) of the Communicable Disease Center, involved the production of film strips with printed texts and recorded narrations on, among other topics, the laboratory diagnosis of tinea capitis in children, ectothrix and endothrix Trichophyton infections, ringworm in animals, blastomycosis, and the slide-culture technique. These strips were supplemented by more than a hundred 2 × 2 inch slides on the histopathology of mycoses and 173 slides of common saprobic moulds (the last produced by Lucille Georg) and a 20-min sound film on coccidioidomycosis (see Ajello, 1957). This material was much used, not only at training courses on various aspects of mycopathology including veterinary mycology in Atlanta, and made a significant educational contribution.

The rest of the world has been less well served. In Europe the most important course is that at the Pasteur Institute in Paris which has been held annually since 1952. This course is spread over five weeks – each session usually comprising an introductory lecture followed by practical work. It is open to French-speaking graduates in medicine, veterinary science, pharmacy, and science and is limited to 21 places (seven of which are normally reserved for foreigners). The course is usually oversubscribed. The scope of the course is wide and the staff of the Pasteur Institute is supplemented by outside lecturers – including some drawn from the more than 500 past students of the course. To gain a diploma the student is at intervals during the course subjected to three 'Interrogations'.

At the Centraalbureau voor Schimmelcultures, Baarn, in the Netherlands courses on medical and veterinary mycology have been organized by Dr G. A. de Vries since 1953. The first course was designed for Dutch students but now, like those at the Pasteur Institute and Duke University, the attendance is international. The course is given in early autumn and lasts four 5-day weeks. The bias is towards mycology. Actinomycetes are included but while serological aspects of mycoses are considered there has been no opportunity for practical work on serological techniques.

In the United Kingdom the MRC Medical Mycology Committee for many years made intermittent attempts to stimulate interest in mycopathological education and it was largely as a result of these efforts that the late Ian Murray, director of the Mycological Laboratory of the Public Health Laboratory Service, arranged the first open fee-paying 10-day summer course on medical mycology at the London School of Hygiene in 1962. The course followed similar lines to those at Duke University and the Pasteur Institute with lectures or demonstrations followed by practical work to which several members of the Medical Mycology Committee

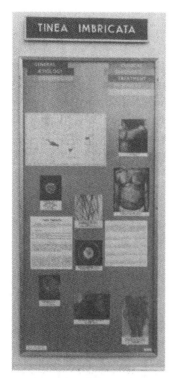
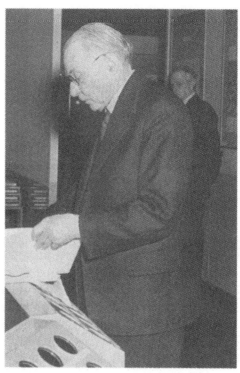

Fig. 51. Mycoses Section of the Wellcome Museum of Medical Science.
A, one of the screens; B, Sir Archibald Gray opening the Section,
9 April 1953. (C. L. Bozman, director of the Museum, in the
background).

contributed. The course was a success (as were later courses on the same
pattern) and in 1976 (and since) Murray's example was followed by Dr
E. G. V. Evans of the Mycology Unit of the General Infirmary Leeds. A
complementary innovation has been the course of lectures for clinicians
and medical microbiologists on 'Medicine and Mycology' held in
Cambridge by Dr S. O. B. Roberts – first in 1974 and subsequently repeated. This residential course comprised an intensive series of lectures given
by a range of specialists over a period of 2–3 days and, bench space not
being a limiting factor, the attendance of between 50 and 70 has been
higher than that possible for a course offering practical work.

Another postwar innovation was the addition to the Wellcome Museum
of Medical Science in London of a section on fungus diseases assembled
with the help of Professor Juan Mackinnon and others and formally

opened in 1953 by Sir Archibald Gray, chairman of the MRC Medical Mycology Committee (Fig. 51).

Textbooks, monographs, periodicals

Textbooks

An important prerequisite for training mycopathologists is suitable textbooks. Up to the First World War mycopathology was dominated by interest in ringworm and there were a number of nineteenth-century texts devoted to this topic. In Britain, *Ringworm in the light of recent research,* 1898, by the dermatologist Malcolm Morris was a notable book while Sabouraud's *Les teignes,* 1910, is still a landmark in the history of mycology. So too is the impressive monograph on sporotrichosis by de Beurmann and Gougerot published two years later. Such books were for specialists and were unsuitable as introductory texts.

During the inter-war years in Great Britain medical mycology was dominated by Professor Aldo Castellani, a flamboyant personality and prolific investigator, who became head of a Department of Tropical Mycoses at the London School of Hygiene & Tropical Medicine. It was the third (1919) edition of Castellani & Chalmers *Manual of tropical medicine* (first published in 1910) which was most consulted by those seeking help in matters medical mycological. The most popular alternative up to the mid-nineteen-thirties was the current edition of Brumpt's *Précis de parasitologie,* first published in 1910. Then, in 1935, Carroll W. Dodge's *Medical mycology* appeared. This book is biased towards medical fungi, as were several slighter books published on the continent of Europe during the first quarter of the twentieth century, and, as has been often remarked, is difficult to use but it still remains a valuable reference source on account of the wide scope and accuracy of its extensive documentation.

The breakthrough occurred in 1944 on the publication of the *Manual of Medical Mycology* by the mycologist N. F. Conant and his medical and bacteriological colleagues D. S. Martin, D. T. Smith, R. D. Baker, and J. L. Callaway at Duke University, North Carolina (Fig. 52). This text – one of the Military Medical Manuals of the National Research Council – provided for the first time a concise and balanced account of mycotic disease in man in which, by and large, the mycology was acceptable to mycologists, the clinical aspects to medical men, and the major systemic mycoses were set in perspective.

The book proved a best seller. Its usefulness was confirmed by the call

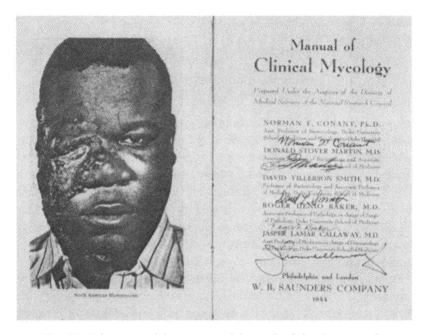

Fig. 52. Title-page and frontispiece of the textbook by Conant *et al.*, 1944.

for additional printings and further editions and it has been flattered by providing the pattern for several other excellent texts by later authors including those of Emmons, Binford & Utz (1963) and Rippon (1982). Important general texts were also published in Brazil by Almeida (1939) and, later, da Silva Lacaz (1967). Atlases and guides to techniques, a selection of which is included in the Bibliography, have also proved popular.

Monographs

Since its inception mycopathology, in marked contrast to phytopathology, has been characterized by the production of book-length monographs on the major diseases. Before 1900 there was Vandyke Carter's account of mycetoma (1874) and in 1897 two French monographs on aspergillosis, by the veterinarian Lucet and the medical pathologist Rénon, appeared almost simultaneously. This century, in addition to the monographs on ringworm and sporotrichosis already mentioned, there was Pallin's account of epizootic lymphangitis in horses (1904) and during the past fifty years cryptococcosis and histoplasmosis have each been monographed twice and candidosis three times.

There have also been books on actinomycosis, coccidioidomycosis, dermatophilosis, and adiaspiromycosis and one up-dating mycetoma (see analysis of the Bibliography).

Periodicals

Although the current periodical literature includes two to three thousand items on mycopathology annually, scattered through several hundred publications, there are few periodicals devoted exclusively to mycopathology. The three most important are the German *Mykosen* (begun in 1957), the *Journal of Medical and Veterinary Mycology* (1962–85 as *Sabouraudia*) which is the official organ of the International Society for Human and Animal Mycology, and the *Review of Medical and Veterinary Mycology* (1943–), a quarterly journal of abstracts compiled at the Commonwealth Mycological Institute and incorporated in the Commonwealth Agricultural Bureaux computerized data base.

Culture collections

Every mycopathological laboratory maintains a collection of fungus cultures relevant to its current research and teaching commitments. In many countries these are supplemented by larger national collections which, like for example the Centraal Bureau voor Schimmelcultures, Baarn, Netherlands, the American Type Culture Collection, Washington, DC, and the Institute for Fermentation Culture Collection, Osaka, Japan, are of international status and play an important rôle as sources of mycological reference material. It is not unusual for national culture collections of micro-organisms to delegate fungi pathogenic for man and higher animals to specialist laboratories such as the Mycology Unit of the Pasteur Institute in France and, in the UK, the Mycological Reference Laboratory of the Public Health Laboratory Service instead of, as formerly, the National Collection of Type Cultures which originated at the Lister Institute, London.

10

Regional developments

As should be clear from the preceding chapters, effective study of mycopathology began in Europe during the first half of the nineteenth century. In the early years of the twentieth century it spread to North America, from where much of the inspiration for developments in this field has originated during the last fifty years. The first developments in Africa and Asia tended to 'follow the flag', that is, workers on secondment from Europe and North America have typically been responsible for the initiation of mycopathological studies in the countries coming within their homelands' spheres of influence. Today there is notable mycopathological activity in Japan, India, South America, and Australasia in parallel with that of North America and Europe. In the review which follows regional developments are sketched in a roughly chronological sequence.

Europe

The science of medical mycology had its origin in France and Germany during the fifth decade of the nineteenth century, particularly in Paris and Berlin, the two leading medical centres of the time. This development, founded on the elucidation of the aetiology of ringworm and thrush, was outlined in Chapters 2 and 4. The interest in mycoses stimulated in **France** at that time has been maintained, in varying intensity, to the present day. Merely to list the names of French workers who have distinguished themselves in this field since the discoveries of Gruby is to epitomize the history of the subject. On the medical side there have been Robin, Duclaux, de Beurmann, Blanchard, Vuillemin, Rénon, Matrouchet, Sabouraud, Bodin, Pinoy, Langeron, Brumpt, Guilliermond, Gougerot, Sartory, Rivalier (all born in the nineteenth century), and the three names associated with the Mycology Unit (founded by Pinoy in 1913) of the Pasteur Institute for the last thirty years, the mycologists Segretain and Mariat, and the medically qualified Drouhet (Fig. 53); on the veterinary side, Mégin, Nocard, Lucet, and Nevue-Lemaire. The more important contributions of

150

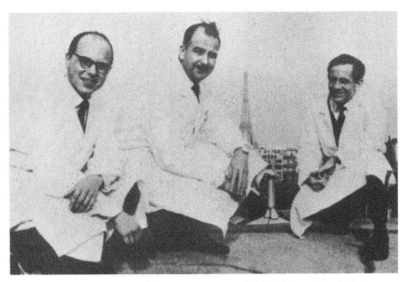

Fig. 53. Emile Drouhet, François Mariat, and Gabriel Segretain (left to right) on the roof of the Laboratoire de Mycologie, Institut Pasteur, Paris, 1954, with the Eiffel Tower in the background.

most of these workers have already been touched on in greater or less detail and so need not be recalled here but the outstanding influence of Sabouraud must again be emphasized. From the turn of the century up to the First World War in almost every country of Europe and North and South America investigations on dermatophytes and other aspects of medical mycology may be traced to workers who studied in Paris with Sabouraud or to students they trained. One important development must not, however, be forgotten; that was the formation of the Société Française de Mycologie Médicale in 1954 with Professor Emile Rivalier (Fig. 54) (Sabouraud's successor at the Laboratoire des Teignes, Hôpital St Louis) as its first president. Its regular meetings and journal (*Bulletin de la Société française de Mycologie médicale*) have done much to promote and maintain interest in mycopathology in France and elsewhere.

Mycetism due to eating poisonous mushrooms has been widely reported in Europe for centuries but no country has generated a larger literature on the subject than France (see Dujuarric de la Rivière & Heim, 1938, and Chapter 8).

In **Germany** Schoenlein, Remak, and B. Langenbeck, all of Berlin, were contemporaries of Gruby and all contributed to an understanding of the aetiology of ringworm and thrush (see Chapter 2). During the rest of the

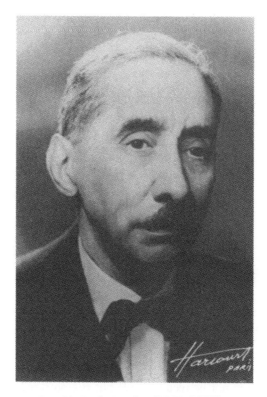

Fig. 54. Emile Rivalier (1892–1979).

century while many German and German-speaking medical men made important contributions on mycotic disease the impression is left that these were usually incidental to the authors' main interest (possibly, in part, the result of war between France and Germany) although the dermatologist H. C. Plaut of Hamburg should perhaps be singled out for his deeper interest in dermatophyte infections in which Jadssohn and Alexander specialized during the nineteen-twenties and thirties (see Plaut, 1903–28). More recently a number of Germans have contributed to the modern movement and in 1961 the Deutschsprachige Mycologische Gesellschaft was formed, with Dr H. Gotz of Essen as the first president, and it adopted the periodical *Mykosen* (1957–) as its official journal. In the veterinary field, the 1874 text by Professor Zürn of Leipzig was innovatory.

Italy has a long and distinguished tradition both for mycology in general and for the recognition and differentiation of fungi pathogenic for plants and animals. In 1729 Pier Antonio Micheli [1679–1737], director of the public gardens at Florence, published his *Nova plantarum genera* which

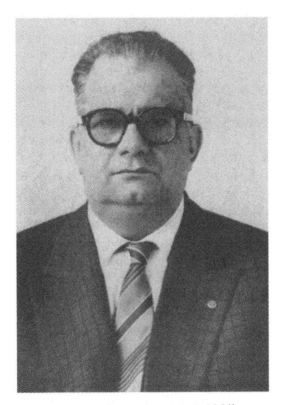

Fig. 55. Raffaele Ciferri (1897–1964).

marked the starting point for mycology as a science. In 1766–7 Felice Fontana [1730–1805] and Giovanni Targioni-Tozzetti [1712–83] independently elucidated the aetiology of wheat rust and in 1835 Agostino Bassi [1773–1856] of Lodi, by elegant experimentation, established the mycotic nature of the muscardine disease of silkworms, the first such infection in animals to be proved. Later the pathogen was named *Botrytis* (now *Beauveria*) *bassiana* in his honour by his fellow countryman G. G. Balsamo-Crivelli [1800–74]. Two other specific epithets well known to mycopathologists and of nineteenth-century Italian origin are (*Histoplasma*) *farciminosum* Rivolta, 1873, and (*Cryptococcus*) *neoformans* Sanfelice, 1895. A notable Italian discovery during the first quarter of the present century was Nannizzi's (1927) of the perfect state of *Microsporum gypseum* although the finding was treated with some scepticism for more than twenty years (see Chapter 2).

Post Second World War mycopathology in Italy was dominated by Piero

Redaelli (professor of pathology at Milan) (Fig. 17) and Raffaele Ciferri (professor of botany at Pavia) (Fig. 55) particularly through the Centro di Micologia Umano e Comparata they founded at the University of Pavia and from which during its first quinquenium some sixty contributions were published including Redaelli's *Le granulomatosi fungine dell'uomo nelle zone tropicali e subtropicale* (see Redaelli & Ciferri, 1943). These authors' *Bibliographia mycopathologica*, 1958, in spite of its inaccuracies, is a most useful source book and Ciferri's two-volume textbook of 1960 was another significant work.

In the **United Kingdom** J. H. Bennett in Edinburgh was among the first to confirm and extend Gruby's findings (Chapter 2). During the second half of the nineteenth century a succession of dermatologists including the two Fox brothers (Tilbury and Colcott), George Thin, MacCall Anderson, and Aldersmith kept an interest in the mycology of the dermatophytes alive and prepared for the flowering that occurred at the turn of the century when Colcott Fox, Blaxall, Adamson, and Malcolm Morris among others led British medical mycology into the van of the advancing movement initiated by Sabouraud. As the twentieth century progressed this initiative was largely lost and the standard of medical mycology fell to a low level during the inter-war years when Castellani (Fig. 20) was the dominating figure (see Chapter 4). Veterinary mycology was more backward. Most attention to mycoses of animals was at first paid to actinomycosis (lumpy jaw) of cattle and among the Board of Agriculture's first 200 advisory Leaflets only two were on mycological topics – No. 67, Favus or white comb in poultry, 1901 and No. 95, Ringworm in cattle, 1903.

The modern revival can be traced back to two men – E. J. Butler and J. T. Duncan. In 1920 Dr Butler – a plant pathologist by profession but medically trained – became the first director of the Imperial Bureau of Mycology set up to abstract the world literature on plant pathology in the monthly *Review of Applied Mycology*. Butler paid increasing attention to medical mycology in this *Review*, which was somewhat incongruous in a periodical designed for plant pathologists (who at that time were widely designated 'mycologists'), and in 1942 a study of the policy of the Imperial Mycological Institute (as the Bureau had become) resulted in consultation with the Medical Research Council on the question of abstracting the medical mycological literature. It was decided that the best way to meet the need was by a separate publication and the first issue of an annual *Annotated Bibliography of Medical Mycology* appeared in 1944. This developed into the quarterly *Review of Medical and Veterinary Mycology* which was at first a joint product of the Bureau of Hygiene & Tropical Medicine, the Imperial Bureau of Animal Health at Weybridge, and IMI. At the same time the MRC established its own Medical Mycology Committee composed of dermatologists, medical pathologists, and non-medical mycologists (who had all practised as plant pathologists) with J. T. Duncan (Fig. 48) (see Ainsworth, 1978) as chairman. During the war, Duncan, lecturer in bacteriology at the London School of Hygiene & Tropical Medicine where he had developed an interest in fungi, was seconded to take charge of the Winchester Laboratory of the newly created Public Health Laboratory Service from where he made a survey of the mycoses of the country (Duncan, 1945). After the war he became head of a permanent Mycological Reference Laboratory established within the PHLS and based at the LSHTM. These developments coincided with, and were stimulated by, the arrival in the country of the first copies of the textbook on medical mycology (Fig. 52) by Norman Conant and his colleagues at Duke University, North Carolina. In 1947, the MRC Committee, re–organized under the chairmanship of Sir Archibald Gray, a London dermatologist and University administrator, attempted the regulation of nomenclature to assure a common language and later arranged a series of annual residential meetings at which medical and veterinary clinicians and pathologists and non-medically trained mycologists all involved to some degree in the practice of mycopathology met one another with increasing confidence. These meetings still continue as one of the main activities of the British Society for Mycopathology. This increased interest in medical mycology was reflected in the establishment of posts for medical mycologists at Leeds, Glasgow, Bristol and other centres including the Commonwealth Mycological Institute; Jacqueline Walker (née Duncan) being the first non-medically qualified mycologist in the country to be appointed to an official post when she joined the Mycological Reference Laboratory of the PHLS as assistant to her father to whose position she eventually succeeded.

The main development in the veterinary field resulted from a two-year survey (sponsored by the Agricultural Research Council) of fungi associated with disease in farm animals carried out by Ainsworth and Austwick in collaboration with the regional veterinary investigation officers of the Ministry of Agriculture (Ainsworth & Austwick, 1955). This led to the establishment of a mycological unit at the Central Veterinary Laboratory, Weybridge, with Austwick in charge. Later Christine Dawson was appointed mycologist at the Veterinary School of the University of Glasgow.

Mycopathology was advanced in Northern Ireland by the creation in 1959 at the Department of Microbiology of Queen's University, Belfast, of a Mycological Diagnostic Laboratory in the charge of D. W. R. Mackenzie[1]

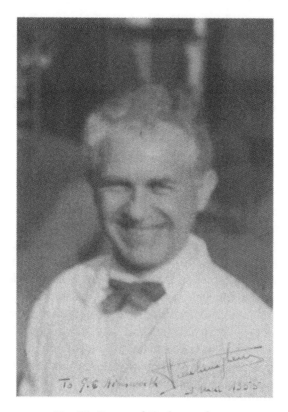

Fig. 56. Raymond Vanbreuseghem.

who is currently head of the Mycological Reference Laboratory of the PHLS of England and Wales.

Other European countries have made important contributions to myco-pathology. In **Sweden** (the homeland not only of Linnaeus but of Elias Fries who with the expatriate Dutchman, Christiaan Hendrik Persoon, living in Paris laid the main foundation of taxonomic mycology) Fredrik Theodor Berg, who had studied in Paris under Gruby, in 1841 independently discovered the nature of thrush. His contemporary Henrik Malmsten proposed the genus *Trichophyton* in 1845. The many contributions made by the Scandinavian countries and **Finland** from 1841 to 1941 have been reviewed by Paldrok (1960). During 1907–37 in **Denmark** the dermatol-ogist Henrik Bang published a number of papers on aspects of the dermatophytes and in the eighteen-eighties E. C. Hansen at the Carlsberg Laboratories, Copenhagen, developed the techniques for discriminating yeasts which were subsequently extended, standardized, and exploited by workers in the **Netherlands** in the laboratory of Kluyver at Delft which has today resulted in the latest edition of *The Yeasts* edited by Kreiger-van Rij. In 1952 a section for fungi of medical importance was established under G. A. De Vries at the Centraalbureau voor Schimmelcultures, Baarn,[2] for diagnostic work and research.

Gedoelst's 1902 textbook on fungi pathogenic for man and animals was a landmark. Recent mycopathology in **Belgium** has been dominated by the investigations of Raymond Vanbreuseghem (Fig. 56) and his school at the Institut de Médecine Tropicale Prince Leopold, Antwerp, which have had repercussions worldwide. Raymond Vanbreuseghem, a dermatologist by training, developed an interest in fungi, studied under Langeron (the second edition of whose textbook he edited), and then engaged in diverse mycopathological investigations, both temperate and tropical, travelled widely and did indefatigable missionary work for mycopathology.

In **Switzerland** Bruno Bloch of Basel made a number of investigations on dermatophytoses, especially the 'id' reaction (see Chapter 5) and recently H. J. Scholer of the Hoffmann-La Roche Company of Basel has published on mucormycosis and its causal agents, aspergillosis, and historical aspects of mycopathology (Scholer, 1974).

Contributions from the Iberian Peninsula have for the most part provided additional records for the dermatophyte flora of Europe. Carneiro (1950) briefly reviewed a decade of mycopathological work in **Portugal** where studies by N. van Uden of the Gulbenkian Institute of Science, Oeiras, Lisbon, on yeasts including the intestinal flora of domesticated animals broke interesting new ground (van Uden *et al.*, 1958). Mycological investigations in **Spain** began late and one of its roots can be traced back to Sabouraud. After the Spanish Civil War (1936–9) Manuel Pereiro Miguens set up a mycological laboratory in connexion with the dermatological clinic at Santiago di Compostela of his father who had studied under Sabouraud at the St Louis hospital in Paris. Later, after a decade in Buenos Aires working with Pablo Negroni, Pereiro Miguens returned to Spain and took over his father's practice while maintaining his mycological interests and in 1984 became president of the Asociación Espãnola de Especialistas en Micologia which had been founded in 1977 (see Miguens, 1984*a*, *b*). For the past three decades he has provided a Spanish presence at many international mycopathological meetings.

There was little nineteenth-century mycopathological interest in the **USSR** and since then dermatophyte infections and candidosis, together with actinomycosis, have attracted most attention. Kashkin's (1959) review of mycopathological publications during the decade 1946–56 provides a typical sample of the Russian output in this field during the postwar period, with one exception. An outstanding feature of twentieth-century Russian work missing from Kashkin's review is that on mycotoxicoses (see Chapter 8), a special interest of A. K. Sarkisov (Fig. 45) at the All Union Institute of Experimental Veterinary Medicine in Moscow where he and others have investigated various aspects of veterinary mycology. About 1970 a Department of Deep Mycoses was set up at the Martzinovsky Institute of Medical Mycology & Tropical Medicine, Moscow, and in 1974 there was an English translation of the 1970 edition of the general mycopathological textbook by Sheklakov (see Sheklakov & Milich, 1974) head of the Department of Mycology of the USSR Ministry of Health's Central Research Institute of Dermatology and Venereal Disease, Moscow.

North America

During the second half of the nineteenth century interest in mycotic disease of man and animals in the United States was slight. Ringworm and candidosis were familiar and in 1886 William Osler recorded a case of human actinomycosis. At the turn of the century American dermatologists visited Sabouraud in Europe and in 1902 Mewborn, a New York dermatologist, independently described and named the cat ringworm fungus (see Chapter 3). Gilchrist reported the first case of blastomycosis in 1896, the sporotrichosis pathogen was first differentiated by Schenck (1898) and Rixford & Gilchrist (1896) and Monbreun (1934) recognized the fungal nature of coccidioidomycosis and histoplasmosis, respectively. In the nineteen-twenties Baily K. Ashford in Puerto Rico played a rather similar rôle to that of Castellani in pre-First World War days in Sri Lanka by investigating candidosis and sprue. The major systemic mycoses were at first considered rare. Between 1905 and 1945 only some 70 cases of histoplasmosis had been recorded worldwide. Ten years later the incidence of histoplasmosis in the United States was estimated in tens of millions (see Chapter 5). This startling change resulted from the recognition of mild to subclinical infections. A parallel case was that of coccidioidomycosis in dry western states where asymptomatic pulmonary infection had been established in 1936–7 (see Chapter 5). These findings greatly stimulated American interest in mycotic disease and for the first time clinical research was given adequate official mycological support.

As indicated in the previous Chapter, the dermatologist J. Gardner Hopkins was the first to employ a trained mycological assistant by recruiting Rhoda Benham to his staff in 1926. Within ten years two other key mycological appointments followed: those of Conant to the Duke University Medical School and of Emmons to the Institute of Health as the first federal medical mycologist.

Norman Francis Conant (Fig. 50), frustrated on financial grounds from embarking on a medical career, after gaining a first degree at Bates College in Maine trained as a mycologist under Professor W. H. Weston (famed as a mycological teacher) at Harvard University where he also came under the influence of C. W. Dodge. On attaining a doctorate (for a study on *Microsporum*; Conant, 1936–7) he was awarded the Sheldon Travelling Fellowship by Harvard and studied in Paris under Langeron and Sabouraud and on his return home accepted an appointment as mycologist in the Bacteriology Department at Duke University, Durham, North Carolina, where apart from a period of war service he remained until his retirement in 1974 and became an international figure for his research, teaching (see Chapter 9), and service on numerous national and international committees.

Chester Wilson Emmons (Fig. 13) on the completion of studies on the genus Penicillium for a doctorate at Columbia University under Professor Robert Harper (another outstanding mycological teacher) with no idea of specializing in medical mycology was, in 1929, enlisted by Gardner Hopkins as the recipient of a five-year grant from the Rockefeller Foundation for research on medical fungi. Emmons thus became a colleague of Rhoda Benham and it was during the tenure of the grant that he completed his classical study on the taxonomy of the dermatophytes (Emmons, 1934) and also contracted a laboratory infection of coccidioidomycosis. In 1934 negotiations began for a position as a federal employee but funds were unavailable until 1936. However, a grant from the College of Physicians & Surgeons enabled Emmons to spend eighteen months in the Dermatology Department of the School of Tropical Medicine, San Juan, Puerto Rico before taking up the post of Senior Mycologist at the National Institute of Health, Bethesda, Washington DC, which was the first federal support for mycology in the United States. Many of Emmons multifarious investigations during the next thirty years have been referred to.

One other federal appointment merits notice. The function of the National Institute of Health (now, for long, the National Institutes of Health) was for fundamental medical research and later the 'Communicable Disease Center' (now the Center for Disease Control) was set up for surveillance studies, etc. and in 1947 Libero Ajello, who like Emmons acquired his mycological training at Columbia University (where his mycological specialization was on chytrids) was appointed to the Center as medical mycologist to work at Duke University with Conant to help him set up a medical mycological facility for the Center. However, shortly after, it was decided to base the mycological centre at Atlanta. Conant was unwilling to leave Duke so Ajello was given the task of developing what is now known as the Division of Mycotic Disease. Another fruitful, and as yet unfinished, career in medical mycology resulted.

The interest in mycopathology in the United States has been widespread during the past fifty years and too many workers have gained prominence for individual treatment. C. W. Dodge has already been mentioned (Chapter 9) and perhaps it is not invidious to recall the names of C. E. Smith of the University of California for his wide-ranging investigations on coccidioidomycosis, M. L. Furcolow of the University of Kansas Medical Center for his studies on histoplasmosis, H. F. Hasenclever for research on *Candida* and candidosis, and, in the veterinary field, L. Z. Saunders of the New York Veterinary College who developed a special interest in mycoses.

In **Canada** notable advances in knowledge of the dermatophytes were made during the mid-thirties by the collaboration of the Winnipeg dermatologist A. M. Davidson with the mycologist Philip Gregory whom Professor A. H. R. Buller had imported from England into his botanical department at Winnipeg to undertake mycopathological research. In 1960, a collection of fungi of medical importance was established at the University of Alberta, Edmonton,[3] with J. W. Carmichael as the curator while from 1952 at McGill University, Montreal (and later Temple University, Philadelphia) Fritz Blank [1914–77] made wide-ranging investigations.

Finally, attention may be drawn to a sociological aspect. At the beginning of this century Erwin F. Smith, plant pathologist and bacteriologist in the United States Department of Agriculture, was among the first to employ women as graduate scientific assistants and during recent years increasing numbers of women have been appointed to posts in medical and veterinary mycology in North America and also throughout the English-speaking world. In the United States there have been Rhoda Benham, Lucille Georg of the Department of Health, who will be remembered for her work on dermatophytes, and, among the living, Charlotte C. Campbell. Eleanor Silver Keeping (née Dowding), a student of Professor Buller's, who began work as mycologist at the Provincial Laboratory of Public Health, Edmonton, Alberta, from where she collaborated with Dr Harold Orr,[4] may be claimed as the first Canadian medical mycologist – although she never attained an official post – and women have done much to advance mycopathology in Great Britain, Australia, and New Zealand.

Central and South America

Notable contributions to medical mycology have emanated from South America, particularly Argentina,[5] Brazil,[6] **Paraguay**[7] and Uruguay. It will be recalled that it was from **Argentina** that coccidioidomycosis was first described in 1892 by Alejandro Posadas, assistant to Professor Roberto Wernicke, and that in 1900 Guillermo Seeber, one of Wernicke's students, reported the first case of rhinosporidiosis. Another eminent worker in Argentina at this time was the French veterinarian J. Lignières who, after training at the Alfort veterinary school, emigrated, to become professor of bacteriology in the Facultad de Agronomia y Veterinaria de Buenos Aires and director of the Instituto Bacteriologico del Ministerio de Agricultura de la Nacion. He is still remembered for his researches with Spitz on anaerobic actiomycetes. The outstanding worker in Argentina during the past fifty years has been Pedro Negroni, director of the Centro de Micologico in the Faculty of Medicine at Buenos Aires and professor of mycology at the University of La Plata who achieved an international reputation for his many and diverse publications (alone and in collaboration) including books on dermatomycoses (1942) and histoplasmosis (1960).

The centre with the longest record of interest in medical mycology in **Brazil** is the Instituto Oswaldo Cruz (founded 1900), sited at Manguinhos near Rio de Janeiro, and renowned for the studies made there by, among others, Paulo Parreiras Horta (on black piedra), Adolpho Lutz (who first described the causal agent of paracoccidioidomycosis), and particularly Olympio Oliveiro da Fonseca [usually known as Olympio da Fonseca filho or O. da Fonseca] [1895–1978] (Fig. 57) and his collaborator Antonio Eugenio de Arêa Lĕao [1895–1971]. Professor da Fonseca who did more than anyone to stimulate mycopathological investigations in Brazil was a parasitologist by training. He developed an interest in fungi and in 1920 the Rockefeller Foundation enabled him to study in the United States, under the mycologists Roland Thaxter (at Harvard University) and Charles Thom and the dermatologist T. C. Gilchrist, and subsequently Europe where he visited the laboratories of Sabouraud, Brumpt, Langeron, and Guilliermond in France and Christine Berkhout in the Netherlands. From 1920 to 1937 he was head of the Section of Medical Mycology of the Instituto Oswaldo Cruz, where he was succeeded by Arêa Lĕao.

Pedro Severiano de Magalhães [1850–1927], professor in the Faculty of Medicine, Rio de Janeiro, was another early Brazilian student of ringworm and other mycoses while later professor Octavio Coelho de Magalhães [1890–1922], his son, made important contributions to the

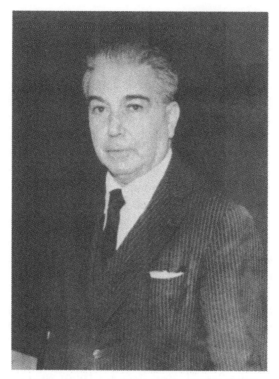

Fig. 57. Olympio da Fonseca filho (1895–1978).

knowledge of mycoses of Minas Gerais, especially by his 'Ensaios de micologia' published in 1935. Mycopathological development in Pernambuco is associated with the name of Jorge de Oliveira Lobo [1900–79] who described the first case of lobomycosis in 1931 in an Indian from the Amazon valley while the versatile mycologist and plant pathologist Professor Augusto Chaves Batista [1916–67], director of the Instituto de Micologia, Recife, also made contributions to the medical mycology of the region.

From the mid-nineteen-thirties major mycopathological developments took place in São Paulo mainly due to the initiative of Floriano de Almeida [1898–1977] who was born and educated in São Paulo where he gained his doctorate of medicine in 1924, came under the influence of da Fonseca, and was later appointed to a chair in the University.

His successor at São Paulo, Carlos da Silva Lacaz, has been equally enthusiastic in promoting mycological studies. Brazilian studies have been dominated by work on paracoccidioidomycosis, widely known as 'South

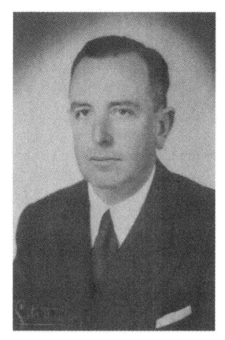

Fig. 58. Juan E. Mackinnon.

American blastomycosis', which was first recognized by Adolpho Lutz in 1908 while director of the Bacteriological Institute of São Paulo before he moved to the Instituto Oswaldo Cruz as director of Medical Zoology. Paracoccidioidomycosis has been the subject of several monographic treatments the latest being the multi-author work edited by Del Negro, Lacaz & Fiorillo (1982). There have also been comprehensive general Brazilian texts by Fonseca (1943), Almeida (1939), and Lacaz; the last, first published in 1967, is currently in its seventh edition.

Veterinary mycology has received less attention since P. S. Magalhães (1883) recorded mouse favus (*Trichophyton quinckeanum*) for Brazil but a number of later records of animal ringworm were summarized by Londero *et al.* (1963).

Two workers are particularly associated with the study of medical mycology in **Uruguay**, which adjoins Brazil and Argentina: Rodolfo V. Talice and Juan E. Mackinnon (Fig. 58), who in succession became Professor of Parasitology at the Instituto de Higiene 'Prof. Arnoldo Berta', Montevideo. After a medical training in Montevideo, Talice studied for two to three years in Paris with Brumpt and Langeron (publishing on yeasts with the latter; Langeron & Talice, 1932) and during the first half of the nineteen-thirties carried out a series of joint investigations on yeasts and a range of other topics with Mackinnon, another Uruguayan, who for the next thirty years retained a lively interest in mycopathology and reported extensive investigations on yeasts, dermatophytes, chromomycosis, mycetomas, and various systemic mycoses including sporotrichosis and its epidemiology (see Chapter 5).

Knowledge of the mycoses of South and Central America has also been deepened by mycopathological activity in **Venezuela,**[8] **Colombia,**[9] and **El Salvador.**[10] Pioneering work on tropical mycoses was undertaken at the School of Tropical Medicine, San Juan, **Puerto Rico** during the nineteen-twenties by Baily K. Ashford on medical yeasts, later by A. L. Carrión on chromomycosis,[12] and because this centre had ties with the Medical School of Columbia University, New York, it was there that Chester Emmons spent a year and a half before 1936 (see above). From 1939 Carroll W. Dodge (a mycologist by training) was, because of his ability to speak Spanish, for a time in Guatemala as an exchange professor in the medical school of the National University (where he did some clinical dermatology) and subsequently he made visits to medical centres in Brazil and Chile (where he was licensed to practise medicine) under the auspices of the Rockefeller Foundation for Medical Research. The outstanding medical mycologist in **Mexico** was A. González Ochoa [d. 1984] and it was from Mexico that recent interest in hallucinogenic fungi stemmed from the explorations of Wasson and Heim (see Chapter 8).

Asia

The first studies on the medical mycology of the Indian subcontinent were made by expatriates. In **India** members of Her Majesty's Indian Medical Service, as exemplified by Vandyke Carter's (1874) investigation of mycetoma in Madras and D. D. Cunningham's (1873) study of the air spora in Bengal, broke new ground. Later in **Sri Lanka** Aldo Castellani made notable discoveries relating to tropical mycoses while working at Colombo as bacteriologist to the Government of Ceylon from 1903 to 1915. The listing of fungi recorded for India is constantly being updated and the census of such records is more nearly complete than for any comparable region.[11] The usual range of fungi pathogenic for animals and man, excluding mycetoma and rhinosporidiosis (the latter monographed by Karunaratne (1964) of Sri Lanka), includes nothing that calls for special comment. Das Gupta et al. (1960) have reviewed Indian medical mycology from its inception to 1959. Mycology was one interest of the School of Tropical Medicine, Calcutta (established 1927), where H. W.

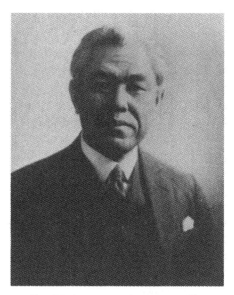

Fig. 59. Masao Ota (1885–1945).

Acton and N. C. Day worked, but during recent times mycological studies have been undertaken by laboratories at Bombay, Lucknow, Jaipur, and New Delhi among others.

Although a late starter, **Japan** currently shows more intense mycopathological activity than anywhere else in Asia. In the nineteen-twenties Professor Masao Ota (Fig. 59) of the Department of Dermatology of the Faculty of Medicine, University of Tokyo, after studying under Professor Langeron in Paris made notable investigations on the dermatophytes (Ota, 1926–8). After the Second World War, in Japan as elsewhere, an increasing number of reports of fungal infections following antibiotic therapy focused attention on fungi as pathogens and in 1952 the Japanese Ministry of Education established the Research Committee of Hyphomycoses (under the chairmanship of Dr Yoshida Takahashi of Juntendo University) and in 1954 this was replaced by the Research Committee of Candidiasis (Chairman Dr Imasato Donomae, Osaka University) which in 1961 published the results of investigations it had instigated (Donomae, 1961). In October 1956 the Japanese Society for Medical Mycology (JSMM) (Iwata, 1977b) was founded with Dr Donomae as the first president and the *Japanese Journal of Medical Mycology* as its journal. At the first annual meeting of the JSMM held at Juntendo University there were about 200 members. In 1984 the individual membership numbered 894.

Part of this growth may possibly be attributed to the strong Japanese interest in mycotoxicoses (see Chapter 9).

A concise review of the mycoses recorded for the **Near** and **Middle East** (Egypt to Saudi Arabia) is that by Mumford (1964).

Africa

The mycoses of Africa have been widely sampled but rarely studied intensively. In 1908, Henry Wellcome established the Tropical Research Laboratories at the Gordon Memorial College at Khartoum in what was then the Anglo-Egyptian Sudan, now **Republic of the Sudan**, supplemented by a laboratory on a steamboat for use on the river Nile. It was here that A. J. Chalmers and R. G. Archibald investigated mycetoma of the Sudan just before and during the First World War and about the same time French workers studied mycetoma of North and West Africa, e.g. Pinoy in Tunisia, Brumpt in Senegal. During the nineteen-thirties Catanei, based at the Institut Pasteur de Algérie, made extensive studies of ringworm in **Algeria** which were the subject of a monograph (Catanei, 1933) and the mycoses of **Madagascar** were investigated by Brygoo (1961) from the Institut Pasteur de Madagascar. E. C. Smith contributed to the knowledge of the mycopathology of **Nigeria** while workers from Belgium have clarified the position in the **Congo**, especially Van Sagehem, who first recognized dermatophilosis in cattle, and Vanbreuseghem who in 1955 summarized his many and diverse investigations on the mycoses of the region. The most notorious outbreak of a mycosis in **South Africa** is the epidemic of sporotrichosis among miners of the Witwatersrand (see Chapter 5). Other mycoses of the region as observed at the South African Institute for Medical Research, Johannesburg have been briefly reviewed by Lurie (1955) and D. G. Steyn, Veterinary Research Officer at Onderspoort, in 1933 drew attention to the potentialities of fungi to produce mycotoxins (see Chapter 8).

Australasia

The first important contribution from **Australia** was Cox and Tolhurst's 1946 monograph on cryptococcosis (*Cryptococcus neoformans*) (as 'human torulosis' caused by *Torula histolytica*) based on the histories of thirteen previously unpublished cases encountered at Alfred Hospital, Melbourne, since 1936. It was, however, the North Shore Hospital in Sydney that became the centre for medical mycology in Australia from a small beginning in 1949 when a few live cultures of fungi pathogenic for man were brought to the Department of Bacteriology by the honorary research assistant Shirley Brown who during the next four years in collaboration with the chief bacteriologist, Beatrix Durie (an Australian by birth), examined a thousand specimens from cases at the hospital for fungi (Durie & Brown, 1953). Largely due to Dr Durie's enthusiasm the mycological work flourished. In 1954 a grant from the National Health & Medical Research Council of Australia enabled Dorothea Frey (doctor of science of the University of Vienna) to be instated as a full-time research-worker; in 1968 she and Durie reported on fungal infections of the skin in Australia, and in 1970 on the deep mycoses. The mycological unit remained incorporated in the Department of Bacteriology until the retirement of Dr Durie in 1964 when it became independent and in the following year the laboratory was designated the National Reference Laboratory in Medical Mycology by the NHMRCA with Dr Frey as Principal Mycologist and Curator. On the veterinary side Connole & Johnston (1967) reviewed their own and others' work on the animal mycoses of Australia.

In **New Zealand** the beginnings of modern medical mycological studies are particularly associated with Mary J. Marples who after education at Bradford and Oxford emigrated to New Zealand where she qualified in medicine and subsequently became professor of microbiology at Otago University, Dunedin. Her interest in medical mycology began during her medical training when her children developed tinea capitis and were excluded from school and this influenced both her choice of topic for a thesis in her final year and her future research interests. In addition to investigations on the incidence and epidemiology of ringworm in New Zealand she also made surveys of skin diseases of Samoa and other Pacific Islands and of New Guinea (see Ajello, 1972) and studies on candidosis in collaboration with Margaret Di Menna whom she introduced to medical mycology and who specialized on yeasts.

In 1974 a Mycological Reference Laboratory was set up at the National Health Institute, Wellington, under F. M. Rush-Munro who, on his retirement in 1980 was succeeded by his former assistant A. J. Woodyer.

J. M. B. Smith (1968) of Otago University, in the light of his own investigations, reviewed animal mycoses in New Zealand where a feature of veterinary studies has been the recognition of facial eczema in sheep and cattle as a mycotoxicosis caused by *Pithomyces chartarum* (see Chapter 8).

POSTSCRIPT

In conclusion, and in part to summarize this introductory historical survey of mycopathology, it is instructive to contrast two standard North American texts bearing the same title – *Medical Mycology* – by Caroll W. Dodge (Missouri Botanical Garden and Henry Shaw School of Botany, Washington University, St Louis) and John W. Rippon (Pritzker School of Medicine, University of Chicago), published in 1935 and 1982, respectively, forty-seven years apart, by two authors of similar background and objective. Both were trained as mycologists, both gained extensive clinical experience of mycoses in Latin America, and the main intention of both was to survey the current state of the art in the light of investigations during the preceding fifty years.

Copies of these two texts have stood side by side on my shelves within arm's reach during the writing of the present book. They are heavy volumes. Each weighs more than two kilogrammes. The former has 900 pages, 142 numbered text-figures, and more than 4000 references; the latter 842 pages (with the text in double columns), more than 500 figures, and 3000 references. There the similarity almost ends and the subtitles (see Fig. 60) would be more appropriate if transposed. Dodge heavily emphasized the fungi (all but three figures (of dermatophytes infecting hairs) are line drawings illustrating the morphology of fungi or actino-mycetes) and reference to clinical aspects of mycoses seems almost incidental while although Rippon certainly gives illustrated description of the pathogens the emphasis is on the diseases for each of which a balanced summary of the aetiology, pathology, epidemiology, clinical features, and therapy is provided. Comparison of the two volumes suggests that medical mycology was revolutionized during the intervening half century, if the use of such an expression is still meaningful. The 'revolution' does not meet the criteria recently laid down by I. B. Cohen in his *Revolution in science*, 1985. The underlying revolution in Cohen's sense occurred a hundred years before when the concept of pathogenicity of micro-organisms, initiated by the experimental demonstrations that fungi were

MEDICAL MYCOLOGY

FUNGOUS DISEASES OF MEN AND
OTHER MAMMALS

BY

CARROLL WILLIAM DODGE, Ph.D.
MYCOLOGIST, MISSOURI BOTANICAL GARDEN ; PROFESSOR, HENRY SHAW SCHOOL OF BOTANY,
WASHINGTON UNIVERSITY
ST. LOUIS

ILLUSTRATED

LONDON
HENRY KIMPTON
263 HIGH HOLBORN, W. C. 1.
1936

JOHN WILLARD RIPPON, Ph.D.
Associate Professor of Medicine
The Pritzker School of Medicine
The University of Chicago
Chicago, Illinois

Second Edition

Medical Mycology

The Pathogenic Fungi
and
The Pathogenic Actinomycetes

W. B. SAUNDERS COMPANY   1982
Philadelphia London Toronto Mexico City Rio de Janeiro Sydney Tokyo

Fig. 60. Title-pages of textbooks by Carroll W. Dodge and John W. Rippon.

able to cause disease in plants, insects, and man, became generally accepted, and concurrently, spontaneous generation and heterogenesis rejected. The marked and rapid deepening, or maturation, in the understanding and practice of mycopathology has been largely the result of the joint application of specialist knowledge and techniques by mycologists, pathologists, medical clinicians, and veterinarians to a neglected field. This quickly yielded spectacular results. Dodge, looking back from the nineteen-thirties, struggled to taxonomize the many fungi which had been reported – frequently on slender evidence – to be causally related to disease in man and higher animals and he accepted more than 600 taxa. Rippon from his standpoint in the nineteen-eighties had a wealth of material on which to draw. He was able to incorporate in his review a taxonomy of the pathogenic fungi which had benefited from among others, advances in knowledge of imperfect fungi and yeast, pleomorphism and dimorphism, and speciation based on morphological criteria which together have reduced the established pathogenic fungi satisfying Koch's postulates to less than two hundred. Rippon's book is also, as he himself recognized, a direct descendant of the classic Duke University text of 1945 developed as one result of the American war effort. Both books are period pieces.

To forecast developments in science is always hazardous but it does appear that the rate of change in mycopathology during the next half century is likely to be less spectacular. It now seems clear that few, if any, fungi are dependent for survival on their pathogenicity for man or higher animals and, on the other hand, equally clear that many fungi are potential or 'opportunistic' pathogens ever ready to take advantage of factors which lower resistance of the host to infection. These last include saprobes so widely distributed in the environment that the elimination of diseases such as histoplasmosis and coccidioidomycosis seems unlikely. Knowledge of such diseases will deepen and improved therapeutic procedures be devised. Other mycoses not yet recognized will be defined while changes in life style or the management of domestic and farm animals, or changes in medical and veterinary practice will provide opportunity for the intervention of potential fungal pathogens. The overall picture of the 'natural history' of mycoses has already been sketched in. There is, however, much scope for increased understanding of the pathogen/host interaction at the cellular and molecular levels which currently lags behind that in plant pathology and bacteriology and the final outcome of such developments is impossible to foresee.

NOTES ON THE TEXT

1. Introduction

1. This collaboration is reflected in the average number of authors per research publication. In the bibliography of this book the numbers are: before 1910, 1.1; after 1960, 2.1.
2. Stran *et al.* (1972).
3. In French *muguet* [lily-of-the-valley, *Convallaria majalis*], a name introduced by Martinet of the Paris Children's Hospital, 1740; German, *Soor*; Swedish, *Torsk*.
4. Loeb transl. **3**: 257.
5. *Ibid.* **3**: 179.
6. According to *The Oxford English Dictionary* the first use of tinea in English was in 1495; the anglicized 'rynge-worm' dating from *c*. 1425.
7. J. Aubry, *Natural history of Wiltshire*, 1847:37. London.
8. W. Dampier, *A new voyage round the world*, edn 7, 1729 [1937 reprint]: 228–9, London.
9. See T. E. Cone, *Am.J.Dis.Child.* **112**: 378–80 (1966).
10. See L. Goldman, *Arch.Derm.Syph.Chicago* **98**: 660–1 (1968); **101**: 688 (1970). (1970).
11. *Veterinarian* **47**: 792 (1984).
12. Bulloch (1938): 217–30.
13. See W. J. Nickerson & J. W. Williams in Nickerson (1947): 130–56 (Chap. 9).
14. *Trans.Br.mycol.Soc.* **30**: 40–1 (1948).
15. L. Ajello in Al-Doory (1977); 294.

2. Aetiology: dermatophytes and the taxonomic problem

1. *Le Dr Gruby, notes et souvenirs* by L. le Leu [who was Gruby's secretary from 1885], 1908, Paris; Kisch (1954): 193–226.
2. Kisch (1954): 213.
3. Kisch (1954): 220; Le Leu, *loc. cit.*: 165.
4. Gruby on 'la vraie teigne' (favus):

   I. Pour reconnaître la vraie teigne, on n'a qu'à la soumettre au microscope; pour cela on se sert d'une petite parcelle de la croûte, délayée avec une goutte d'eau pure; on la met entre deux lames de verre, et on l'examine sous un grossissement linéaire de 300. On y verra une grande quantité de corpuscules ronds ou oblongs, dont le diamètre longitudinal est de 1/300 à 1/100 de millim., et le transversal de 1/300 à 1/150 de millim.; ils sont transparents, à bord net, à surface lisse, incolores, légèrement jaunâtres et composés d'une seule substance. On remarque en outre de petits filaments articulés d'un diamètre de 1/1000 à 1/250 de millim., transparents et incolores; la forme générale de ces filaments est cylindrique ou ramifiée, selon la partie de la croûte à laquelle ils appartiennent.

Les filaments cylindriques sont composés de corpuscules oblongs ou ronds, qui ont souvent l'aspect d'un chapelet; les filaments ramifiés, au contraire, sont munis de distance en distance de cloisons végétales, représentant des cellules oblongues, dans lesquelles on trouve de petites molécules rondes et transparentes d'un diamètre de 1/10000 à 1/1000 de millim. Quelquefois on trouve des granules adhérentes aux filaments, pareilles aux spores de la *Tortula olivacea* et *T. Sachari*, présentées dans l'ouvrage intitulé: *Icones fungorum* de M. Corda (Pragæ, 1841, tome IV). La forme de ces filaments met leur caractère végétal hors de doute; elles appartiennent au groupe des mycodermes, selon M. Brongniart.

Comme nous n'avons pas encore trouvé une molécule de la vraie teigne qui ne soit chargée d'un grand nombre de ces mycodermes, celles-ci constituent un vrai charactère essentiel de cette maladie. (Gruby (1841): 73–4).

5. See Kisch (1954): 227–96; Seeliger (1985).
6. Gruby on 'mentagre' (tinea barbae; ectothrix trichophytosis):

On peut facilement distinguer les trois espèces de cryptogames de la teigne faveuse, du muguet et de la mentagre, aux caractères suivants:

Dans les porrigophytes (cryptogames de la teigne faveuse),

1°. Les cryptogames se logent entre les cellules d'épiderme;
2°. Ils descendent sur les follicules du poil;
3°. Ils sont enfermés dans des capsules propres;
4°. Ils n'ont que très-rarement de granules dans leurs tiges;
5°. Leurs sporules sont grands et ordinairement ovales.

Dans les aphthaphytes (cryptogames du muguet),

1°. Les cryptogames sont logés entre les cellules d'epithelium;
2°. Ils forment des champignons;
3°. Leurs branches se détachent de la tige selon des angles aigus;
4°. Les branches sont rarement striées.
(Gruby (1842b): 513).

Dans les mentagrophytes (cryptogames de la mentagre),

1°. Les cryptogames logent entre le poil et sa gaîne;
2°. Ils remontent de la racine du poil vers l'epiderme;
3°. Ils n'ont point de capsules;
4°. Ils ont presque toujours des granules dans leurs tiges;
5°. Leurs sporules sont petits et ordinairement ronds.

Dans les mentagropytes (cryptogames de la mentagre),

1°. Les cryptogames sont logés dans les gaînes du poil;
2°. Ils ne forment point de champignons;
3°. Leurs branches se détachent selon des angles de 40 à 80°;
4°. Leurs branches sont toujours striées.

7. Gruby on 'porrigo decalvans' (microsporosis):

Les sporules garnissent la surface externe de la gaîne, et se pressent les unes contre les autres au même niveau; cependant on en rencontre quelques-unes à la surface des cheveux, adhérentes aux branches. Les sporules sont ordinairement rondes; il y en a aussi quelques unes d'ovales: leur diamètre est de 1/1000 à 5/1000 de millimètre. Les sporules ovales sont un peu plus grandes; elles ont de 2/1000 à 5/1000 sur 4/1000 à 8/1000 de millimètre de diamètre. Elles sont transparentes, ne contiennent point de molécules dans leur intérieur, et dans l'eau elles se gonflent.

J'appellerai ces cryptogames, à cause de la petitesse de ces sporules, *Microsporum*; et, pour attacher à cette partie nouvelle de la Pathologie le nom de ce célèbre académicien qui, par ses belles recherches sur la muscardine, a beaucoup contribué à diriger les esprits sur les plantes parasites qui détruisent les tissus vivants des animaux, je propose le nom de *Microsporum Audouini*, pour dénoter les individus végétaux qui constituent le Porrigo decalvans.

Le tissu du poil est altéré par la quantité de *Microsporum Audouini* qui se fixe à sa surface. D'abord le cheveu devient opaque à l'endroit où les cryptogames sont placés; sa surface lisse devient rugueuse. L'épithelium qui tapisse la surface des cheveux perd son éclat et sal cohésion; il tombe peu à peu. Le tissu des cheveux lui-même devient friable, cassant; un tel cheveu casse même par la simple flexion, et de là partout où les plantes parasites ont envahi le tissu de cheveux: les cheveux tombent peu à peu jusqu'à ce qu'il n'en reste aucune trace. L'endroit où les cheveux sont tombés est d'un blanc grisâtre, parce qu'il y a encore une quantité de cryptogrames qui reste à la surface de l'épiderme dont les cellules sont devenues le siège.

Outre ces cryptogames, on n'y rencontre aucun produit pathologique, ni inflammation, ni vésicules, ni pustules, ni hypertrophie de l'épiderme. Cette maladie de la peau doit donc être placée dans la nouvelle classe des *maladies parasitiques végétales*, c'est-à-dire dans la nouvelle classe de maladies que j'ai nommée *phytoparasites*, à côté de la *teigne faveuse*, de la *phytomentagre* et du *muguet*.

Les microspores d'Audouin, qui constituent la *phytoalopécie* (c'est le nom par lequel je propose de distinguer cette affection), ont beaucoup d'analogie avec les cryptogames qui constituent la maladie que j'ai décrite sous le nom de *phytomentagre*; mais ils se distinguent surtout par le siège. Les cryptogames, dans la mentagre, sont placés dans les follicules des poils, et même autour de leurs racines; les microspores d'Audouin, au contraire, sont placés autour de la partie aérienne des cheveux. Les sporules, dans le microspore d'Audouin, sont plus petites, ses branches plus courtes que dans les mentagrophytes.
Gruby (1843): 302.

8. Gruby on 'teigne tondante' (endothrix trichophytosis):

Les cryptogames qui constituent la teigne tondante diffèrent tellement de ceux qui constituent la phyto-alopécie, qu'il est impossible de confondre ces deux maladies. Leur siège même, leur développement et le rapport qu'ils offrent avec le tissu des cheveux, diffèrent également de celui de la phyto-alopécie.

D'abord les cryptogames de la teigne toudante ne sont formés que de sporules en chapelet; rarement on voit des sporules allongées imitant des branches.

Les cryptogames de la phyto-alopécie, au contraire, ont de nombreuses branches courbées, ondulées, et les sporules placées à leur côte.

Dans la teigne tondante, les sporules sont grandes; leur diamètre varie de 2 à 6 sur 4 à 8 millièmes de millimètre.

Les sporules des cryptogames de la phyto-alopécie, au contraire, sont extrêmement petites; leur diamètre n'est que de 1 à 5 millièmes de millimètre, et c'est aussi pour cela que je les ai appelées *Microsporon*.

Dans la teigne tondante, les sporules remplissent l'intériur des cheveux, tandis que leur surface externe est peu changée.

Les sporules de *Microsporon Audouini*, au contraire, sont placées à la surface externe des cheveux, et forment une véritable gaîne autour d'eux.

Les cryptogames de la teigne tondante prennent naissance et se développent dans la racine des cheveux.

Le *Microsporon Audouini*, au contraire, se développe à la surface externe des cheveux, en dehors des follicules.

Ces caractères sont tellement constants dans la teigne tondante, qu'il n'y a pas un seul cheveu malade dans cette affection qui ne les présente.

La teigne tondante résulte uniquement du développement des cryptogames que nous avons déjà décrits, et elle mérite par conséquent d'être classée parmi les maladies dues à des parasites végétaux, à côté de la *phyto alopécie*, de la *mentagrophite*, de la *porrigophite* et de l'*aphtophite*.

Et pour distinguer la teigne tondante de la phyto-alopécie, je propose de donner à c'ette dernière la dénomination de *rizo-phyto-alopécie*. Gruby (1844*a*): 585.

9. M. J. Berkeley, *Introduction to cryptogamic botany*, 1857: 299. London.
10. Obituary: L. M. Pautrier, *Ann.derm.Syph.Paris*, 7e sèr., 9: 275–97 (1938).
11. Emmons on the generic classification of dermatophytes:

There appear to be three natural groups of dermatophytes: 1. There are species of Trichophyton which reproduce in culture principally by subspherical to clavate conidia and also form in many if not all species smooth, thin-walled, few-celled, clavate macroconidia. In hairs infected by species of Trichophyton the arthrospores into which the hyphae become cut are more or less definitely in rows. There are three subgroups, according to clinical manifestations, which coincide roughly with three types of Trichophyton cultures.

2. The second group comprises Epidermophyton with at least one distinct species, Epidermophyton floccosum (Epidermophyton inguinale), which reproduces in culture exclusively by oval to egg-shaped macroconidia which are smooth and thick-walled, with from two to a few cells. Clinically, an infection by Epidermophyton cannot always be distinguished from an infection by Trichophyton, but as the former occurs in typical lesions in the axillae and in the groin it is a definite clinical entity. It does not invade the hair. Species of Endodermophyton and some species of Trichophyton which are ordinarily found on the glabrous skin invade the hair, however, in experimentally infected guinea-pigs...

3. There are finally species of Microsporum which reproduce in culture principally by spindle-shaped macroconidia (except in M. Audouini and its varieties in which the macroconidia are few and abortive) and also produce clavate conidia. In hairs infected by species of Microsporum there is a

characteristic sheath around the hair in which the arthrospores are arranged as in a mosaic.

In this enumeration favus and its causal fungus have, so far, been omitted. Common favus is caused by one species which has been called Achorion Schoenleinii.[21a] Infection by this fungus usually causes a definite clinical picture. However, some of the clinical features of favus may be caused by other fungi. As Sabouraud has pointed out, the fungi which occasionally cause favus show affinities with species of Microsporum of animal origin and with endothrix species of Trichophyton. A. Schoenleini is mycologically a species of Trichophyton. The classification is simplified by omitting the generic name Achorion. The principal species, A. Schoenleini then becomes T. Schoenleini, and the others fall into their respective groups. This step ends the confusion arising in cases such as that in which the same fungus is called A. gypseum when it is isolated from a favus-like lesion, and Microsporum fulvum when it comes from another type. This step is recommended by Langeron and Milochevitch.[6] The generic name Endodermophyton is likewise discarded because its species are referable to the Trichophyton group.

There appear to be adequate reasons for accepting these three genera and excluding others.
(Emmons (1934): 356–7).

3. Names: problems of nomenclature

1. See Ainsworth (1978); also Chapter 10.
2. *International nomenclature of diseases*, vol 2, *Infectious diseases*. Part 2. *Mycoses*, xii + 47 pp. (1982). Geneva.
3. See J. E. Mackinnon, *Sabouraudia* **1**: 3–7 (1961).
4. Nomenclature of mycoses, *Sabouraudia* **18**: 78–84 (1980). German version, W. Loeffler, *Mykosen* **26**: 346–84 (1983).

4. Problems of pathogenic status with special reference to mycelial yeasts

1. *Br.J.Derm.Syph.* **50**: 516 (1938).
2. See *Lancet 1849* **2**: 493.
3. *Report of the thirty-eighth meeting of the British Association for the Advancement of Science...* Notices and abstracts: 83–7, 1869.
4. There have been two major summaries of the literature on Candida and candidosis, by Winner & Hurley (1964) and Odds (1979), each with more than two thousand references, to which the report on a symposium on Candida infections held in 1965 (Winner & Hurley, 1966) and the reviews by Skinner (1947) and Hurley (1967) are useful supplements.
5. *Arch.Physiol.norm.path.* **1**: 290–305 (1868).
6. W. Zopf, *Die Pilze* (Breslau): 478 (1890).
7. A method devised by M. W. Beijerinck in 1889 and modified by Lodder in *Die anaskosporogenen Hefen* (1934) and Langeron (1945): 484.
8. There have been many surveys of the incidence of Candida at all sites and

selections have been tabulated and summarized by Skinner (1947), Winner & Hurley (1964), and Odds (1979).

9. See P. K. C. Austwick *et al.* in Winner & Hurley (1966): 89–100.
10. For example Emmons, Binford & Utz (1963), edn 2 (1970): 258.
11. See Ainsworth & Austwick (1957), edn 2 (1971): 74–6.
12. Ainsworth, *Rep.Commonw.mycol.Conf.* **6**: 7–22, 1961; *Sabouraudia* **5**: 81–6 (1966).

5. Epidemiological problems

1. F. Desenne, *C.R.Acad.Sci.Paris* **87**: 34–6 (1878); M. A. Morris, *Trans.path.Soc.* **30**: 441–4 (1879); E. Juhel-Renay, *Ann.Derm.Syph.Paris* **2**:777–85 (1888); **3**:765–72 (1890); G. Behrend, *Arch.Derm.Syph.* **23**:994–5 (1891).
2. In a case reported by Moyer & Keeler (1964), an albino tribesman on a Panama offshore island who was a 'therapeutic chanter' had encouraged the growth of black piedra by not oiling his hair, as was the custom, and sleeping with his head on the soil so that his hair was completely blackened by the fungus.
3. Ajello (1957):78.
4. See *Rev.med.vet.Mycol.* **2**:2073 (1957); Balows (1971).
5. Dimorphism has been reviewed by A. H. Romano in Ainsworth & Sussman (eds), *The fungi* **2**:181–209 (1966); and G. T. Cole & Y. Nozawa in Cole & Kendrick (eds), *Biology of conidial fungi* **1**:97–133 (1981).
6. See preceding note.
7. See *J. Bact.* **84**:829–40, 841–58 (1962); *Biochim.Biophys.Acta* **58**:102–19; **64**:548–51 (1962).
8. See T. Benedek, *Mycopathologia* **16**:104–6 (1962) on the history of hairbaiting.
9. See L. C. Sutthill & Campbell, *Sabouraudia* **4**:1–2 (1965); R. P. Tewari & Campbell, *ibid.* **4**:17–22 (1965).
10. See M. L. Dillon in Al-Doory (1977):165–7.

6. Therapeutic problems

1. Loeb transl. **3**: 257.
2. Bohn edn **5**: 334.
3. *Ibid.* **4**: 226–7.
4. J. W. Churchman (*J.exp.Med.* **16**: 221 (1912)) showed gentian violet to inhibit the growth of certain Gram+ bacteria and D. L. Farley (*Arch.Derm.Syph. Chicago* **2**: 1459–65 (1920)) incorporated gentian violet (1:250000) in agar media to facilitate the isolation of dermatophytes.
5. Küchenmeister (1857): 259 writes:

   'Küchler...at Darmsadt...in spite of pitch-plaster...has experienced two relapses. That this extremely energetic physician did not, perhaps, proceed mildly in the application of pitch-plaster, the following will show. I give this account because it indicates particularly the preparation and application of the pitch-plaster. One takes ordinary, not thin, cobblers' wax, and places it not too thickly on strong, not too fine, not too new, not too smooth, nor very heavy linen, with the addition of a few drops of turpentine. After the most thorough removal of the hair possible, as far as it goes, and after removal of the crust which becomes softened by the oil, the pitch-plaster is placed on the diseased part, over all the space implicated. The plaster for two or three finger-breadths near its anterior border should be kept free from pitch and turned over, by which it can be better taken hold of and pulled off. Incisions also should be made round the edges of the plaster, by which it fits closer, but not too deep by which it is pulled off afterwards. The pitch remains on eight days, and is then removed. The patient is seated on a stool without a back or crosswise, and his head and neck made fast sideways under the plaster by the grasp of a strong assistant. A second assistant at the head stands behind the patient, with his eight fingers on the fore part of the slightly loosened plaster, places his knee on the neck of the patient, and draws off, if possible, the whole plaster with a haul. This proceeding has sometimes to be gone over again. The stench on the removal is often horrible. The part never remains bare.

Küchler saw relapses twice; still he has not specified altogether the number of cases. On removal once all the pitch remained on the diseased part, because the assistant had taken very strong linen. Küchler ordered a smoothing iron to be heated, and better linen ironed on. With such faults, and such heroic *corrigentia*, who would not admire the pitch-cap treatment!

6. Küchenmeister (1957): 184.
7. *Br.J.Derm.Syph.* **61**: 7–8, 1949.
8. A. R. Martin, *Vet.Rec.* **70**: 1232 (1958) reported that a similar result had been noted at the Research Laboratories of Imperial Chemical Industries Ltd, in 1956 and in November 1957 a Polish team at Poznan claimed successful treatment of human ringworm with salicylhydroxamic acid *per os* (J. Alkiewicz *et al.*, *Nature* **180**: 1204–5, (1957)).
9. See *Arch.Derm. Chicago* **81**: 649–882 (1960).
10. *Wall Street Journal*, 6 March 1968, fide Ajello in Al-Doory (1977): 294.
11. See Baldwin (1981).
12. *Iodine Facts.* **1**, 56 (1940–6).
13. See H. Lechevalier *et al.*, *Mycologia* **45**: 155–71 (1953).
14. See *Rev.med.vet.Mycol.* **2**, 1436.
15. *Ibid.* **2**, 1430.
16. *Ibid.* **3**, 1010.
17. *Ibid.* **3**, 945.
18. *Ibid.* **4**, 948.
19. Both British and Irish Circulars and Orders are reprinted in Pallin (1904): i–xxiii.

7. Spores as allergens: a problem of sensitization

1. *C.R.Acad.Sci.Paris* **50**: 748–52 (1860).
2. *Monthly microscop.J.* **5**: 45–9 (1870).
3. K. R. May, *J.sci.Instrum.* **22**: 187–95 (1945).
4. For a summary see Hyde (1972).
5. See Storm van Leeuwen (1924) and Van der Werf (1958) for bibliography.
6. Also for haemostasis in horses by E. G. La Fosse, 'Maréchal des petites Ecuries du Roi', 1768, fide Smithcors (1958): 268, 280, pl. 32.
7. Eliasson (1982): 441.

8. R. Fawcett, *Br.J.Radiol.* 9: 172–95 (1936); 11: 378–92 (1938).
9. E. Törnell, *Acta tuberc.Scand.* 20: 212–35 (1946).

8. Mycetism, myxotoxicoses, and hallucinogenic fungi: toxicological problems

1. See Houghton (1885): 40. During the present century English-speaking mycologists, due to deficiencies in their classical education, have, with or without acknowledgement, usually obtained their information on references to fungi in the Greek and Roman classics from the compilation by the Rev. William Houghton, Rector of Preston, Wellington, Shropshire, published in 1885, supplemented by Buller (1915) who was assisted by his schoolmaster friend the amateur mycologist W. B. Grove, an able classical scholar.
2. Houghton (1885): 24.
3. *Ibid*: 29–30.
4. *Ibid*: 40.
5. Joanne H. Phillips, *Actes xxviiie Congr.Internat.d'Hist.Med.* (Paris, 1982): 204.
6. *Satires* ii, 4, 20.
7. Ford & Clark (1914): 79.
8. G. Watson, *Theriac and mithridatium*, 165 pp. (1966) (London; Wellcome Hist.Med. Libr.).
9. C. D. Badham, *A treatise of the esculent funguses of England*, 1847 (p. viii), prints an English translation of the regulations introduced in 1837 for the sale of fungi in the Rome market. The provisions include that:

   ...all the Funguses brought into Rome by the different gates should be registered...a certain spot should be fixed upon for the Fungus market, and that nobody under penalty of fine and imprisonment should hawk them about the streets...at seven o'clock, A.M., precisely, the Inspector should pay his daily visit, and examine the whole, the contents of the baskets being previously emptied on the ground...the stale Funguses of the preceding day, as well as those that were mouldy, bruised, filled with maggots, or dangerous...should be sent under escort and thrown into the Tiber...the Inspector should be empowered to fine or imprison all those refractory to the above regulations...
10. Dujarric de la Rivière & Heim (1938): 51–2.
11. J. M. Bauchet, *Bull.Br.mycol.Soc.* 17: 110–1 (1983).
12. There have been a number of books on mycotoxicoses – for a selection see analysis of the Bibliography – also many symposia which have frequently subsequently appeared as books, e.g. G. N. Wogan (ed.), *Mycotoxins in foodstuffs*, 1965 (Cambridge, Mass; MIT Press); I. F. H. Purchase (ed.), *Mycotoxins in human health*, 1971 (London); J. V. Rodricks (ed.), *Mycotoxins and other fungal related food problems*, 1976 (Washington, DC; Am.chem.Soc.).
13. D. Atanasoff, *Ergot of grains and grasses*, 127 pp. (305 refs), 1920 (BPI US Dep.Agric.); Barger (1931); Sarkisov (1954); Bové (1970).
14. See Ainsworth (1976): 186–8 for details.
15. Bové (1970): 136.
16. Ibid.: 138.
17. Ibid.: 141.

18. Garrison (1929): 186; Bové (1970): 147; Backman (1952): 295.
19. 'Ignus sacra' of Lucretius [95–55 BC] was thought by Barger (1930) to have been erysipelas.
20. Linnaeus, *Dissertationes Academicae*, De Raphania. Resp. G. Rothman, 1763, Upsala.
21. See Ainsworth & Austwick (1957): 107–8.
22. Kathleen Sampson & J. H. Western, *Diseases of British grasses and herbage legumes*, edn 2 (1948) (Cambridge): 45.
23. See the comprehensive reviews by Mayer (1953); Forgacs & Carll (1962): 347–58, A. Z. Joffe in Ciegler *et al.* (1971–2) 7: 139–89, and Wyllie & Morehouse (1977–8) 3: 21–86.
24. See Forgacs & Carll (1962): 278–93; Forgacs in Ciegler *et al.* (1971–2) 8: 95–128; E. L. Hintikka in Wyllie & Morehouse (1977–8) 2: 152–61 (horses), 3: 87–9 (man).
25. See K. Uraguchi, *J.Stored Prod.Res.* 5: 227–36; also in Ciegler *et al.* (1971–2) 6: 637–80.
26. See P. M. Scott in Wyllie & Morehouse (1977–8) 1: 318–20.
27. See the reviews by C. P. McMeckan, *Endeavour* 3: 89–96 (1961); J. F. Filmer, *N.Z. J.Agric.* 97: 202–9 (1958); *Span* 4: 112–16 (1961).
28. *The variation of plants and animals under domestication* 2: 337 (1868) (London). Reprinted in Ainsworth (1976): 191.
29. E. A. Ellis, Mycol.Papers 76 (1960).
30. B. S. James, *Nature* 184: 1327 (1957).
31. Maureen E. Lacey & P. H. Gregory, *Nature* 193: 85 (1962).
32. Blount (1961).
33. F. D. Asplin & R. B. A. Carnaghan, *Vet.Rec.* 73: 1215–19 (1961).
34. R. M. Loosemore & L. M. Markson, *Vet.Rec.* 73: 813–14 (1961).
35. J. D. J. Harding, *Vet.Rec.* 73: 1362.
36. Lancaster *et al.* (1961); Schoental (1961).
37. Ruth Alcroft & R. B. A. Carnaghan, *Vet.Rec.* 74: 863–4 (1962).
38. P. K. C. Austwick in Wyllie & Morehouse (1977–8) 2: 279–301; Austwick & Ayerst (1963).
39. Anon. *Vet.Rec.* 72: 710 (1960).
40. Blount (1961).
41. Also R. O. Sinnuber & J. H. Wales in Wyllie & Morehouse (1977–8) 2: 489–95.
42. J. V. Rodricks in Wyllie & Morehouse (1977–8) 3: 161–71.
43. Wyllie & Morehouse (1977–8) 2: 297.
44. In the *Review of Medical and Veterinary Mycology* for 1984 more than 225.
45. Goldblatt (1969); Heathcote & Hibbert (1978).
46. Including W. H. Butler in Purchase (1974): 1–28, 145 refs.
47. See also L. D. Scheel in Wyllie & Morehouse (1977–8) 2: 121–42.
48. See P. Krog in Wyllie & Morehouse (1977–8) 2: 236–56.
49. For references, mostly in Japanese, see Wyllie & Morehouse (1977–8) 1: 341–2.
50. E. B. Smalley in Wyllie & Morehouse (1977–8) 1: 449–57; 2: 111–20.
51. Wasson (1968).
52. Lowy (1972).
53. R. E. Schultes, *Bot.Mus.Leafl. Harvard Univ.* 7: 37–54 (1939).
54. R. G. Wasson, *Life* (International edn) 10 June 1957: 44–60.
55. R. E. Young, R. Milroy, S. Hutchison & C. M. Kesson, *Lancet 1982* 1: 213–15.

9. Training mycopathologists: an educational problem

1. This Chapter is, in part, based on the First Ian Murray Memorial Lecture read to the British Society for Mycopathology, 21 March 1978.

10. Regional developments

1. See *Ulster med.J.* **29**: 70–3 (1960); **30**: 29–30 (1961); **31**: 93–4 (1962).
2. See K. B. Raper, *Mycologia* **49**: 884–92 (1957).
3. *Catalogue of the University of Alberta mold herbarium and culture collection. First edn. 56 pp. 1966. Edmonton, Alberta.*
4. See E. Silver Keeping, *Can.med.Ass.J.* **68**: 386–7 (1953).
5. See Negroni (1939).
6. See Lacaz (1982).
7. See Recalde (1980).
8. See Campins (1958).
9. See Restrepo-Moreno *et al.* (1962).
10. See Bloch *et al.* (1975).
11. See E. J. Butler & G. R. Bisby, *The fungi of India*, 1931; revised to 1952, by R. S. Vasudeva (1960); also later supplements.
12. See A. L. Carrión & Margarita Silva in Nickerson (1947): 20–62.

BIBLIOGRAPHY & CHRONOLOGY

In addition to publications cited in the text the bibliography includes references to publications on the history of mycopathology (*) and representative mycopathological texts.

The names of mycoses, pathogens, etc. in **bold face** type are first or significant records, not all of which are referred to in the text.

History

General: dermatophytes (Sabouraud, 1910; Ajello, 1977*a*); farmer's lung (Eliasson, 1982); favus (Alkiewicz, 1967; Seeliger, 1985); fungal allergy (Cunningham, 1873; Van der Werff, 1958; Gregory, 1973); hallucinogenic fungi (Wasson, 1957, 1968; Lowy, 1972); mycetism (Houghton, 1885; Grmek, 1982); mycetoma (Carter, 1874; Sran *et al.*, 1972); mycotoxicoses (Mayer, 1953; Hesseltine, 1979); paracoccidioidomycosis (Ajello, 1972*b*); systemic mycoses (Scholer, 1974); thrush (Higgs, 1973). See also Emmons (1940). Rippon (1982) has useful historical summaries of the principal mycoses.

Regional: Argentina (Negroni, 1939); Brazil (Lacaz, 1983); Germany (Hornstein, 1981; Schadewalt, 1981); India (Randhawa *et al.*, 1961); Japan (Iwata, 1977); Paraguay (Recalde, 1980); Portugal (Carneiro, 1950); Spain (Pereiro Miguens, 1984); UK (Ainsworth, 1951, 1978).

Bibliography: Lindau & Sydow (1908–17); Ciferri & Redaelli (1958); O'Meara & Wheelwright (1971), avian mycoses; Ainsworth & Stockdale (1983); *Review of Medical and Veterinary Mycology*, 1944–.

Biography: Ainsworth & Stockdale (1984); Kisch (1954); Schwarz & Baum (1965); Baldwin (1981); Huntington (1985).

Bacteriology: Bulloch (1938).

Dermatology: Gray (1951).

Medicine: Garrison (1929).

Mycology: Ainsworth (1976).

Veterinary Medicine: Smithcors (1957).

Representative mycopathological textbooks, monographs, etc.

General texts:

Medical: Robin (1853), Küchenmeister (1857), Hallier (1866), Bodin (1902), Gedoelst (1902, 1911), Guéguen (1904), Castellani & Chalmers (1910), Brumpt (1910–49), Sartory (1920–23), Neveu-Lemaire (1921), Castellani (1927–8), Henrici (1930), Vuillemin (1931), Jacobson (1932), Nannizzi (1934), Dodge (1935), Lewis & Hopper (1939), Conant et al. (1944), Ciferri (1960), Emmons et al. (1963), Zapater (1965), Lacaz (1967), Sheklakov & Milich (1974), Kashkin & Sheklakov (1978), Rippon (1982), Howard (1983–5).

Veterinary: Robin (1853), Zörn (1874), Gedoelst (1902, 1911), Guéguen (1904), Neumann (1892) Nevue-Lemaire (1911), Curasson (1942), Ainsworth & Austwick (1959), Jelínek & Sobra (1961), Jungerman & Schwartzman (1972).

Atlasses: Moss & McQuown (1953), Vanbreuseghem (1966), Frey et al. (1979), Salfelder et al. (1979), Chandler et al. (1980), McGinnis et al. (1982).

Clinical: Warnock & Richardson (1982), Roberts et al. (1984).

Epidemiology: Chick et al. (1975), Al-Doory (1977), Klastersky (1982), Warnock & Richardson (1982), DiSalvo (1983).

Methods: Sartory (1924), Redaelli (1931), Hazen & Reed (1955), Zapater (1956), Beneke (1957), Segretain et al. (1960), Ajello et al. (1962), McGinnis (1980).

Serology: Seeliger (1963), Evans (1976), Palmer et al. (1977).

Therapeutics: Speller (1980).

Monographs: actinomycosis (Cope, 1938; Bronner & Bronner, 1969); adiaspiromycosis (Jellison, 1969); allergy (Van der Werff, 1958; Al-Doory & Domson, 1984); aspergillosis (Lucet, 1897; Rénon, 1897; Austwick, 1975); candidosis (Winner & Hurley, 1964, 1966; Hurley, 1967; Odds, 1979; Bodey & Fainstein, 1985); coccidioidomycosis (Fiese, 1958; Ajello, 1977b; Stevens, 1980); chromomycosis (Al-Doory, 1972); cryptococcosis (Cox & Tolhurst, 1946; Littman & Zimmerman, 1956); dermatophytoses (Anderson, 1861; W. T. Fox, 1863; Thin, 1887; Morris, 1898; Sabouraud, 1910; Alexander et al., 1928; Negroni, 1942); epizootic lymphangitis (Pallin, 1904); hallu-cinogenic fungi (Wasson, 1957, 1968; Heim et al., 1958, 1967); histoplasmosis (Negroni, 1960; Sweany, 1960; Ballows, 1971; Domer & Moser, 1980); mycetism (Dujarric de la Rivière & Heim, 1938; Lincoff & Mitchell, 1977; Rumack & Salzman, 1978); mycetoma (Carter, 1874; Negroni, 1954; Mahgoub & Murray, 1973); mycotoxi-coses (Sarkisov, 1954, 1964; Bilaï, 1960; Moreau, 1968; Goldblatt, 1969, aflatoxin; Ciegler et al., 1971–2; Purchase, 1974; Heathcote & Hibbert, 1978, aflatoxin; Wyllie & Morehouse, 1977–78; Ueno, 1983, trichothecenes); paracoccidioidomycosis (Ajello, 1977b; Del Negro et al., 1982); rhinosporidiosis (Karunaratne, 1964); sporotrichosis (de Beurmann & Gougerot, 1912).

Mycoses of the eye (Cavara, 1928); François & Rysselarene, 1972); lungs (D. T. Smith, 1947; Buechner, 1971).

Before 1800

BC

c. 2000–   *Atharva-Veda.* **Mycetoma** of the foot. See Sran *et al.* (1972).
1500

5th   Hippocrates (the Asclepiad of Cos). *Hippocrates with an English*
cent.   *translation* by W. H. S. Jones & E. T. Withington. 4 vols, 1923–31
   (Loeb Classical Libr.). **Thrush**

AD

1st cent. Celsus, Aurelius Cornelius, *De re medicina* [in 8 books.
   Engl. transl. W. G. Spencer, 3 vols, 1935–8 (Loeb Classical Libr.)].
   Thrush, Favus
   Pliny the Elder (Caius Plinius Secundus), *Historia naturalis* [in 37 books.
   Engl. transl., J. Bostock & H. T. Riley, 6 vols, 1856–93 (Bohn's Classical
   Libr.).]

1582   Lonitzer, A. (Lonicerus). *Kreuterbuch*: 285. Frankfurt-
   on-Main. **Ergot**

1658   Bauhin, G. *Theatri botanici.* Liber primus: 434. Basle. **Ergot**
   (figured)

1676   Dodart, D. Lettre de M. Dodart, contenant des choses fort
   remarquables touchant quelques grains. *Mém. Acad.roy.Sci. depuis*
   1666 jusqu'à 1699 **10**: 561–6 (1730).

1698   Floyer, John. *A treatise of the asthma.* London.
1700   Ramazzini, B. *De morbis artificum diatriba.* Modena [Engl.
   transl. Anon. *A treatise of the diseases of tradesmen* (1705). London.]

1748   Arderon, W. The substance of a letter from Mr William
   Arderon F.R.S. to Mr Henry Baker F.R.S. *Phil.Trans.* **45** (487): 321–3.
   Saprolegniosis

1749   Réaumur, R.A.F. de. *Art de faire éclorre et d'élever en toute*
   saison les oiseaux domestiques de toutes espèces...Paris. [*Engl.transl. Anon.*
   The art of hatching and bringing up domestick fowls of all kinds, at any time
   of year (1750) London.]

1771   Rosen von Rosenstein, N. *Underrättelse om Barms Sjuk-domar och Deras*
   Botemedal. Stockholm. [Engl. transl. A. Sparrman. *The diseases of*
   children and their remedies (*1776*). London. Fr.transl., 1778; Ital.,
   1780; Germ., 1785.]

1800

1813   Bateman, T. *A practical synopsis of cutaneous diseases according to the*
   arrangement of Dr Willan, exhibiting a concise view of the diagnostic
   symptoms and the method of treatment. London.
   Montagu, G. *Supplement to the ornithological dictionary (1802).* London.

1815   Mayer, A. C. Verschimmelung (Mucedo) in lebenden Körper.
   Deutsch.Archiv.Physiol. (Meckel's) **1**: 310–12.

1824   Plumbe, S. *A practical treatise on diseases of the skin...*London. [edn
   4 (1857)]

1832   Owen, R. On the anatomy of the flamingo (*Phaenicopteris ruber*, L.).
   Proc.zool. Soc. Lond. **2**: 141–4.

1835   Véron, P. Mémoire sur le muguet. *Arch.gén.Med.* 8: 466. **Candidosis (oesophageal)**

1835–6 Bassi, A. *Del mal del segno, calcinaccio o moscardina...Teoria*, 1835: *Practica*, 1836. Lodi [Facsimile, 1956. Novarra; Engl.transl. of *Teoria*, *Phytopath. Classics* 10 (1958).] **Muscardine disease of silkworms**

1837   Hube, X. *De morbo scrofuloso.* Dissert.inaug. Berlin. [Fide Kisch (1954)]

1839   Langenbeck, B. Auffindung von Pilzen auf der Scheimhaut der Speiseröhre einer Typhus-Leiche. *Neue Not.Geb.Natur-u.-Heilk.* ('Froricep's Notizen') 12 (252) col. 145–7.

        Schoenlein, J. L. Zur Pathogenie der Impetigines. *Arch.Anat.Physiol. wiss.Med.* ('Müller's) *1839*: 82, Taf. iii, fig. 5 **Favus**

1841   Berg, F. T. Torsk i mikroskopiskt anatomiskt hänseende. *Hygiea, Stockholm* 3: 541–50. **Candidosis**

        Gruby, D. (a) Mémoire sur une végétation qui constitue la vrai teigne. *C.R. Acad.Sci.Paris* 13: 72–5. (b) Sur les mycodermes qui constituent la teigne faveuse. *Ibid.* 13: 309–11. [Engl.transl. Zakon & Benedek (1944).]

1842   Bennett, J. H. On the vegetable nature of tinea favosa (Porrigo lupinosa of Bateman) its symptoms, causes, pathology and treatment. *Lond.Edinb. Monthly J.med.Sci.* 2: 504–19.

        Gruby, D. (a) Recherches anatomiques sur une plant cryptogame qui constitue le vrai muguet des enfants. *C.R. Acad.Sci.Paris.* 14: 634–6. (b) Sur une espèce de mentagre contagieuse resultant du développement d'un nouveau cryptogame dans la racine des poils de la barbe de l'homme. *Ibid.* 15: 512–13. [Engl.transl. Zakon & Benedek (1944).]

        Remak, R. Gelungene Impfung des Favus. *Med.Z.* 11: 137.

1843   Gruby, D. Recherches sur la nature, la siége et le développement du porrigo decalvans ou phyto-alopécie. *C.R.Acad.Sci.Paris* 17: 301–3. [Engl.transl. Zakon & Benedek (1944).] **Microsporum audouinii**

1844   Bennett, J. H. On the parasitic fungi found growing in living animals. *Trans.roy.Soc.Edinb.* 15: 277–94. [read 1842.]

        Gruby, D. (a) Recherches sur les cryptogames qui constituent la maladie contagieuse du cuir chevelu décrite sur le nom de teigne tondante (Mahon), herpes tonsurans (Cazenave). *C.R. Acad.Sci.Paris* 18: 583–5. [Engl.transl. Zakon & Benedek (1944).] (b) Note sur les plantes cryptogamiques se Développant en grand masse dans l'estomac d'une malade atteinte, depuis huit ans, de difficultés dans la déglutition des aliments, soit liquides, soit solides. *Ibid.* 18: 586–8.

1845   Lebert, H. *Physiologie pathologique ou recherches cliniques expérimentales et microscopiques sur l'inflamation, la tuberculisation, les tumeurs. la formation de cal, etc.* 2 vols. Paris. [2: 490 **Oidium schoenleini.**]

        Malmsten, P. H. *Trichophyton tonsurans. hårskärande Mögel Bidtrag till utredande af de sjukdomar, som vålla hårets affall.* Stockholm. [Germ. transl. *Arch.Anat.Physiol.wiss.Med.* (Müller's) *1848*: 1–19] **Trichophyton tonsurans**

        Remak, R. *Diagnostische und pathogenetische Untersuchungen in der Klinik* des Geh. Raths Dr Schönlein auf dessen Veranlassung angestellt und mit Benutzung anderweitiger Beobachtungen veröffentlicht. 242 pp. Berlin. **Achorion schoenleini**

1846   Berg, F. T. *Om Torsk hos Barn.* Stockholm. [Germ.transl. (1848), Bremen.] Eichstedt, C. Pilzbildung in der Pityriasis versicolor. *Neue Not.Geb. Natur-u.-Heilk.* ('Froricep's Notizen') Ser. 2, **39** (853): 270–1. **Pityriasis versicolor**

1847   Robin, C. *Des végétaux qui croissent sur l'homme et sur les animaux vivants.* Paris (Thesis Fac.Sci.).

Sluyter, T. *De vegetabilibus organismi animalis parasitis, ac de novo epiphyto in pityriasi versicolore obvio.* Diss. inaug. Berlin [Fide Virchow (1856).] **Aspergillosis (human)**

1848   Tersáncky, J. Die Schimmelräude die Athmungsbeschwerden der Arbeiter in Schwammfabriken. *Oesterr.med.Wochenschr.* **9**: 259.

1849   Wilkinson, J. S. Some remarks upon the development of epiphytes with the description of a new vegetable formation found in connexion with the human uterus. *Lancet 1849* **2**: 448–51. **Candidiosis (vaginal)**

1850

1850–   Fresnius, G. *Beiträge zur Mykologie.* Frankfurt. **Aspergillus fumigatus**
63

1853   Robin, C. *Histoire naturelle des végétaux parasites qui croissent sur l'homme et sur les animaux vivants.* + Atlas of 16 pl. Paris. **Microsporon mentagrophytes, M. furfur, Oidium albicans**

Tulasne, L. R. Mémoire sur l'ergot des glumacées. *Ann.Sci.nat.Paris*, 3 Sér., **20**: 5–56. **Claviceps purpurea**

1855   Küchenmeister, F. *See* 1857.

1856   Virchow, R. Beiträge zur Lehre von den beim Menschen vorkommenden pflanzlichen Parasiten. *Arch.Path.Anat.Physiol.* (Virchow's) **9**: 557–93.

1857   Küchenmeister, F. *On animal and vegetable parasites of the human body.* (Engl.transl. by E. Lancaster of *Die in und an dem Körper des lebenden Menschen vorkommenden Parasiten*, 1855, Leipzig), 2 vols. London. [Vol. 2: 111–271, vegetable parasites.]

1858   Bennett, J. H. *Clinical lectures in the principles and practice of medicine*, edn 2. Edinburgh.

Lowe, J. On the identity of *Achorion schoenleini* and other vegetable parasites with *Aspergillus glaucus. Trans.bot.Soc.Edinb.* **5**: 193–204.

1861   Anderson, T. McCall. *On the parasitic affections of the skin.* London. [edn 2 (1868).]

Pasteur, L. Mémoire sur les corpuscles organisés qui existent dans l'atmosphère. Examen de la doctrine des générations spontanées. *Ann.Sci.nat.Paris* 4è sér., **16**: 5–98.

1861–5 Tulasne, L. R. & C. *Selecta fungorum carpologia*, 3 vols. Paris. [Engl.transl. W. B. Grove, A. H. R. Buller (ed.) (1931) Oxford.]

1862   Salisbury, J. H. (a) Remarks on fungi, with an account of experiments showing the influence of the fungi of wheat-straw, on the human system...*Am.J.med. Sci.* **44**: 17–28. (b) Inoculating the human system with straw fungi, to protect it against contagion of measles: with some additional observations relating to the influence of fungoid growth in producing disease and in the fermentation and putrefaction of organic bodies. *Ibid.* **44**: 387–94.

Zenker, W. Encephalitis mit Pilzentwicklung im Gehirn. *Jahrb.Ges.Natur-u-Heilk.* (Dresden) *1862*: 51–2. **Candidosis (cerebral)**

1863   Berkeley, M. J. The fungus foot of India. *Intellectual Observer Lond.* **2**: 248–57. [See also *J.Linn.Soc.* **8**: 139–42 (1865).]

Fox, W. Tilbury. *Skin diseases of parasitic origin: their nature and treatment.* London.

Michel, M. Action nuisible des Mucédinées qui se developpent sur la canne de Provence altérée. *J.Chem.méd.Pharm. Toxicol.* 4e sér., **9**: 308.

1865   Cohnheim, I. Zwei Fälle von Mykosis der Lungen. *Arch.Path.Anat.* (*Virchow's*) **33**: 157–9. **Aspergillosis (human pulmonary)**

Hallier, E. Die Natur des Favuspilzes und sein Verhältniss zu *Penicillium glaucum* Auct. *Z.Med.Naturwiss.Jena* **2**: 220.

1866   Hallier, E. *Die pflanzlichen Parasiten des menslichen Körpers*...Leipzig.

Salisbury, J. H. On the cause of intermittent and remittent fevers, with investigations which tend to prove that these affections are caused by species of *Palmella*. *Am.J.med.Sci.* **51**: 51–75.

1867   Rabenhorst, G. L. Zwei Parasiten an den todten Haaren der Chignons. *Hedwigia* **6**: 49. **White piedra (*Pleurococcus beigelii*)**

1868   Quinquaud, M. Nouvelles recherches sur le muguet. *Arch.Physiol. norm.path.* **1**: 290–305. ***Syringospora robini***

1869   Schmiederberg, O. & Koppe, B. *Das Muscarin, das giftige Alkaloid des Fliegenpilzes, Agaricus Muscarius L., seine Darstellung...und sein Verhältniss zur Pilzgiftung im allgemeinen.* Leipzig.

Trousseau, A. *Lectures on clinical medicine, delivered at the Hotel-Dieu, Paris.* Transl. from the edn of 1868 by J. R. Cormack, **2**: 618–30 [Lecture xxi, Thrush.] London (New Sydenham Soc.).

1871   Hirt, L. *Die Krankheiten der Arbeiter. I. Die Staubinhalationskrankheiten.* Breslau.

1873   Blackley, C. H. *Experimental researches on the cause and nature of Catarrhus aestivus (hay-fever or hay-asthma).* London. [Facsimile (1959).]

Cunningham, D. D. Microscopic examination of air. 58 pp. 14 pl. Ex *Ninth Annual Rep., Sanitary Commissioner, Government of India, 1872.* Calcutta.

Hogg. J. *Skin diseases, an inquiry into their parasitic origin, and connection with eye infections; also the fungal or germ theory of cholera.* London.

Rivolta, S. *Dei parassiti vegetali come indroduzione allo studio delle malattie parassitaire e delle alterazioni dell'alimento degli animali domestici.* Turin. ***Cryptococcus farciminosus***

1874 Carter, H. V. *On mycetoma or the fungus disease of India*. 118 pp., 11 pl. London.

Zürn, F. A. *Die Schmarotzer auf und in dem Körper unserer Haussäugetiere... II Theil: Pflanzliche Parasiten*. Weimar.

1876 Fürbringer, P. Beobachtungen über Lungenmykose beim Menschen. *Arch.path.Anat.Physiol*. (Virchow's) **66**: 303–65. **Mucormycosis (pulmonary)**

1877 Bollinger, O. Ueber eine neue Pilzkrankheit beim Rinde. *Centralb. med. Wissensch*. **15**: 481–5. **Actinomyces bovis** Harz

Parrot, J. *Clinique des nouveau-nés. L'athrepsie, Leçons recuelliés par le Dr Troisier*. Paris. [Le Muguet, pp. 73–93.]

1878 Smith, W. G. The salmon disease. *Gdnrs' Chron*. **9**: 560–2.

1879 Manson, P. Notes on tinea imbricata, an undescribed species of body ringworm. *China Imp.Maritime Customs, Med.Rep.,Spec.ser.2*, 16th issue: 1–11.

1881 Mégnin, P. Nouvelle maladie parasitaire de la peau chez un coq. *C.R.Soc.biol.Paris* **33** (= sér. 7, **3**): 404–6. **Trichophyton gallinae**
Schmiederberg, O, Bermerkungen über die Muskarinwirkungen. *Arch. exp.Path.Pharm*. **4**: 376.

Thin, G. On *Trichophyton tonsurans* (the fungus of ringworm). *Proc.roy. Soc*. **33**: 234–46.

1882 Huxley, T. H. Saprolegnia in relation to salmon disease. *Quart.J. microscop.Sci*. NS **22**: 311–33.

1883 Magalhães, P. S. Caso de favus em um ratinho. *Gazeta Med.Bahia* **7**: 480–4.

Miquel, P. *Des organismes vivant de l'atmosphère*. Paris (Thèse,Fac.Med.Univ.Paris.)

1885 *Houghton, W. Notices of fungi in Greek and Latin authors. *Ann.Mag.nat.Hist*. Ser. 5, **15**: 22–49, 153–4.

1886 Duclaux, E. Sur le *Trichophyton tonsurans*. *C.R.Soc.Biol.Paris* **38** (= sér. 8,3):14–16.

Osler, W. Actinomycosis. *Med.News, New York* **49**: 443.

1887 Audry, C. Sur l'évolution du champignon du muguet. *Rev.Med*. **7**: 586–95.

Thin, G. *Pathology and treatment of ringworm*. London.

Verujski, D. Recherches sur la morphologie et la biologie du *Trichophyton tonsurans* et de *l'Achorion schoenleini*. *Ann.Inst.Pasteur* **1**: 369–91.

1888 Nocard, E. Note sur la maladie des boefs connue à la Guadeloupe sous nom de farcin. *Ann.Inst.Pasteur* **2**: 293–302. **Farcy of cattle**

1889 Baillon, H. *Traité de botanique médicale cryptogamique*: 234. Paris. **Malassezia furfur**

Trevisan, V. *I generi e le specie delle Bacteriaceae*: 9. Milan. **Nocardia farcinica**

1890 Dieulafoy, G., Chantemesse, A. & Widal, F. Pseudo-tuberculose mycosique des gaveurs de volailles. *Bull. Méd*. **4**: 748

Eppinger, H. Ueber eine neue Pathogene Cladothrix und eine durch sie hervorgenufene Pseudotuberculosis. *Wein.klin. Wochenschr*. **3**: 221–3. **Nocardiosis (human)**

Schmorl, G. Ein Fall von Soormetastase in der Nier. *Zbl.Bact.* 7: 329–35. **Candidosis (disseminated)**

1891   Furthmann, W. & Neebe, C. H. Vier Trichophytonarten. *Monatsch. Prakt.Derm.* 13: 477–88.

Kobert, R. Matières toxiques dans les champignons. *Petersb.med.Wochenschr. 1891*: 51–2.

Sakaki, J. [Toxicological problems on the deteriorated rice infested by fungi.] *J. Tokyo med. Ass.* 5: 1097–104. [In Jap.]

Wolff, M. & Israel, J. Ueber Reincultur des Actinomyces und seine Uebertragbarkeit auf Thiere. *Arch.Path.Anat.Physiol.* (Virchow's) 126: 11–59.

1892   Djélaleddin-Moukhtar. De la trichophytie des régions palmaire et plantaire. *Ann.Derm.Syph.Paris* 3: 885–915. **Tinea pedis**

Neumann, L. G. *Traité des maladies parasitaires non microbiennes des animaux domestiques*, edn 2. Paris.

Posadas [as Posada], A. Ensayo anatomopatológico sobre una neoplasia considerada como micosis fungoidea. *An.Circ.Med. Argent.* 15: 481–97.

Wernicke, R. Über einen Protozoenbefund bei Mycosis fungoides (?). *Zbl.Bakt.* 12: 859–61.] **Coccidioidomycosis**

1892–3 Sabouraud, R. Contribution à l'étude de la trichophytie humaine. Étude clinique, microscopique, et bactériologique sur la pluralité des trichophytons de l'homme. *Ann.Derm.Syph.Paris* sér. 3 3: 1061–87.

Ernst, P. Über eine Nierenmycose und das geichzeitige Vorkommen verschiedner Pilzformen bei Diabetes. *Arch.path. Anat.* (Virchow's) 137: 486–538. **Aspergillosis (kidney)**

1894   Gaucher, E. & Sergent, E. Un cas de pseudotuberculose aspergillaire simple chez un gaveur de pigéons. *Bull.mem.Soc.mèd.Hop.Paris* sér. 3, 11: 512–21.

Vincent, H. Étude sur le parasite du pied de Madura. *Ann.Inst.Pasteur* 8: 129–51. **Streptothrix madurae**

1895   Adamson, H. G. Observations on the parasites of ringworm. *Br.J. Derm.* 7: 202–11, 237–44. **Adamson's fringe.**

Fish, P. A. A histological investigation of two cases of an equine mycosis, with a historical account of a supposed similar disease, called bursattee, occurring in India. *Ann.Rep.U.S. Bur.Pl.Industr.* 12–13: 229–59.

Rénon, L. Deux cas familiaux de tuberculose aspergillaire simple chez des peigneurs de chevaux. *C.R.Soc.biol.Paris* 47(= sér. 10, 12): 694–6.

Sanfelice, F. Sull'azione patogene dei blastomiceti. *Ann.Ist. Igiene R.Univ. Roma* 5: 239–62. **Saccharomyces neoformans**

1896   Blanchard, R. Parasites végétaux à l'exclusion des bactérières. In C. Bouchard, *Traité de pathologie générale* 2: 811–926. **Trichophyton concentricum, Nocardia asteroides**

Gilchrist, T. C. A case of blastomycetic dermatitis in man. *Johns Hopkins Hosp.Rep.* 1: 269–83 **Blastomycosis**

Rixford, E. & Gilchrist, T. C. Two cases of protozoan (coccidioidal) infection of the skin and other organs. *Johns Hopkins Hosp.Rep.* 1: 209–68. *Coccidioides immitis*

1897   Lucet, A. *De l'Aspergillus fumigatus chez animaux domestiques et dans les oeufs en incubation. Étude clinique et expérimentale.* Paris.

Rénon, L. *Étude sur l'aspergillose chez les animaux et chez l'homme.* Paris.

Gilchrist, T. C. & Stokes, W. R. A case of pseudo-lupus caused by Blastomyces. *J.exp.Med.* 3: 53–78. **Blastomyces dermatitidis**

1898   Morris, M. *Ringworm in the light of recent research.* London.

Schenck, B. R. On refractory subcutaneous abscesses caused by a fungus possibly related to the Sporotricha. *Johns Hopkins Hosp.Bull* 9:286–90. **Sporotrichosis**

Third International Congress of Dermatology. 1896. Official Transactions edited by J. T. Pringle. London. [Ringworm and the Trichophytons, pp. xvi, 492–596.]

1899   Matrouchet, L. & Dassonville, C. Sur le champignon de l'herpès (Trichophyton) et les formes voisines et sur la classification des ascomycètes. *Bull Soc.mycol.Fr.* 15: 240–53.

1900

1900   Hektoen, L & Perkins, C. F. Refractory subcutaneous abscesses caused by Sporothrix schenckii, a new pathogenic fungus. *J.exp.Med.* 5: 77–89. **Sporothrix schenckii**

Ophüls, W. & Moffitt, H. C. A new pathogenic mould. (Formerly described as a protozoan: Coccidioides immitis pyogenes.) Preliminary report. *Philad.med.J.* 5: 1471–2. [See also Ophüls (1905).] **Coccidioides immitis.**

Seeber, G. R. *Un neuvo esporozuario parásito del hombre. Dos casos econtrades en pólipos nasales.* Tesis Fac.Méd. Univ.Nat. Buenos Aires. **Rhinosporidiosis**

1902   Bodin, E. *Les champignons parasites de l'homme.* Paris.

Gedoelst, L. *Les champignons parasites de l'homme et des animaux domestiques.* Brussels.

Mewborn, A. D. A case of ringworm of the face and two of the scalp contracted from a Microsporon of the cat with some observations on the identification of the source of the infection in ringworm by means of cultures. *N.Y.med.J.* 76: 843–9.

Neisser, A. Plato's Versuche über die Herstellung und Verwendung von 'Trichophyton'. Nach seinem Ableben mitgeteilt. *Arch.Derm.Syph. Vienna* 60: 63–76.

Plaut, H. C. Züchtung der Trichophytiepilze *in situ. Zbl. Bakt.* 31: 213–21.

1902–4 Lignières, J. & Spitz, G. Contribución à l'étude des affections connues sous le nom d'actinomycose (actinobacillose). *Rev.Soc.Med. Argentina* 10: 5–105 (1902). *Ibid.* 2e mémoire. Actinomycose a Streptothrix (*Streptothrix spitzi*). *Arch.Parasitol.* 7: 428–79.

1903   de Beurmann, L. & Ramond, L. Abcès sous-cutanés multiples d'origin mycosique. *Ann.Derm. Syph.Paris* 4: 678–85.

Haan, J. & Hoogkamer, L. J. Hyphomyces destruens equi. *Arch.Wiss.Prkt. Tierhlk.* 29: 395–410.

Patterson, J. H. *The cause of salmon disease: a bacteriological examination.* Glasgow (Fishery Board for Scotland).

1903–4 O'Kinealy, F. Localised psorospermios of the mucous membrane of the septum nasi. *Proc.laryngol.Soc.London* 10: 109–12; 11: 43–44 (1904).

1903– Plaut, H. C. Die Hyphenpilze oder Eumyceten. In W. Kolle &
28   A. von Wasserman (eds.), *Handbuch der pathogen Microorganismen* 1: 526–660, 1903; Aufl. 2, 5: 1–154 (1913); Aufl. 3,5 (Teil 1)(1928).

1904 Dubendorfer, E. Ein Fall von Onychomycosis-blastomycetica. *Dermatol.Zbl.* 7: 290–302. **Candidosis (onychomycosis).**

Guéguen, F. *Les champignons parasites de l'homme et des animaux.* Paris.

Pallin, W. A. *A treatise on epizootic lymphangitis.* edn 2 (Sept. 1904) [edn. 1 (June 1904).] London.

Sabouraud, R. & Noiré, H. Les teignes cryptogamiques et les rayons X. *Ann.Inst.Pasteur.* 18: 7–25. Traitement des teignes tondantes par les rayons X à l'École Lailler (Hôpital St Louis). *Presse Méd.* 12: 825–7. **X-ray epilation**

1905 Brumpt, E. Sur le mycétome à grains noirs, maladie produite par une mucédinée du genre *Madurella* n.g. *C.R.Soc.Biol.Paris* 58: 997–9. **Madurella**

Hansmann, G. H. Über eine Bischer nicht beobactete Gehirnerkrankung durch Hefen. *Verh.dt.Ges.Path.* 9: 21–4. **Cryptococcosis (cerebral)**

Ophüls, W. Further observations on a pathogenic mould formerly described as a protozoan (*Coccidioides immitis, Coccidioides pyogenes*). *J.exp.Med.* 6: 433–86. Coccidioidal granuloma, *J.Am.med.Ass.* 45: 1291–6 (1905).

1906 Brumpt, E. Les mycétomes. *Arch.Parasitol.* 10: 489–572, 10 pl., 90 refs.

Darling S. T. A protozoön general infection producing pseudotubercles in the lungs and focal necroses in the liver, spleen and lymphnodes. *J.Am.med.Ass.* 46: 1283–5. **Histoplasmosis (*Histoplasma capsulatum*)**

Ford, W. W. The toxins and antitoxins of poisonous mushrooms (*Amanita phalloides*). *J.infect.Dis.* 3: 191–224.

Vincent, H. Sur unicité du parasite de la maladie de Madura (*Streptothrix madurae* H. Vincent) et sur ses formes génératives. *C.R.Soc.Biol.Paris.* 41: 153–5, 216–17.

1907 Hamberger, W. W. A comparative study of four strains of organisms isolated from four cases of generalized blastomycosis. *J.infect.Dis.* 4: 201–9.

Lutz, A. & Splendore, A. Sopri una micosi observata in uomini e topi [*Mus decumanus*]. Contribuzione alla conoscenza delle cosi dette sporotrichosi. *Ann.Ig.Sperim.* 17: 581–666.

1908 de Beurmann, L. & Gougerot, H. Découverte du *Sporotrichum beurmanni* dans la nature. *Bull.Mém.Soc.Med.Hôp.de* Paris sér. 3, 26: 733–8.

Lutz, A. Uma mycose pseudococcídica localizada na bocco e observanda no Brasil. Contribução ao conhecimento das hyphoblastomycoses americanas. *Brasil Med.* 22: 121–4, 141–4. **Paracoccidioidomycosis**

Splendore, A. Sobre a cultura de uma nova especie de cogumelo patho-génica do homen. (*Sporotrichum* Splendore ou '*Sporotrichum asteriodes*' n. sp.) *Revta. Soc. scient.S.Paulo* **3**: 62.

1908– *Lindau, G. & Sydow, P. Thesaurus litteraturae mycologicae et*
17 *lichenologicae.* 5 vols. Leipzig [Krankheits-erreger bei Menschen und Tieren, **5**: 451–524 (1917).]

1909 Adamson, H. G. A simplified method of X-ray application for the cure of ringworm of the scalp: Kienböck's method. *Lancet 1909* **1**: 1378–80.

Carougeau, J. Sur une nouvelle mycose sous-catanée des équidés. *J.méd. vét.Zootechnie* **60**: 8–22, 75–90, 148–153.

Forbes, J. G. A case of mycosis of the tongue and nails in a female child aged 3½ years. *Br.J.Derm.* **21**: 221–3. [Case report.] **Candidosis (chronic mucocutaneous)**

Splendore, A. Sobre un caso de blastomycose generalizada. *Revta Soc. scient.S.Paulo* **4**: 52.

1910 Adamson, H. G. The Metropolitan Asylums Board's school for ringworm. A report on the work there carried out, with special reference to X-ray treatment. *Br.J.Derm.* **22**: 46–9.

Castellani, A. (a) Observations on a new species of *Epidermophyton* found in tinea cruris. *Br.J.Derm.* **22**: 147–50. *Epidermophyton rubrum* (b) Observations on 'tropical broncho-oïdiosis'. *Br.med.J. 1910* **2**: 868–9. *Oidium tropicale*

Castellani, A & Chalmers, A. J. *Manual of tropical medicine.* London & New York. [edn 2 (1913); 3 (1919).]

Hyde, J. N. & Davies, D. J. Sporotrichosis in man with incidental consideration of its relation to mycotic lymphangitis in horses. *J.cutan.Dis.* **28**: 321–52.

Lord, F. T. The etiology of actinomycosis. *J. Am. med. Ass.* **55**: 1261–3. A contribution to the etiology of actinomycosis. *Boston med.surg.J.* **163**: 82–5.

Sabouraud, R. *Les teignes.* Paris. (= *Maladies du cuir chevelu.* III. *Les maladies cryptogamiques.*) [History, pp. 1–90; refs pp. 813–46.]

1910– Brumpt, E. *Précis de parasitologie.* edn 1 (1910); edn 6 (1949).
49 Paris.

1911 Gedoelst, L. *Synopsis de parasitologie de l'homme et des animaux domestiques.* Brussels.

Horta, P. Sobre uma nova forma de piedra. Sur un nouvelle forme de piedra. *Mem.Inst.Oswaldo Cruz* **3**(1): 86–107. **Black piedra**

Nevue-Lemaire, M. *Parasitologie des animaux domestiques. Maladies parasitaires non bactériennes.* Paris.

1912 de Beurmann, L. & Gougerot, H. *Les sporotrichoses.* Paris. **Sporotrichosis**

Castellani, A. Observations on the fungi found in tropical broncho-mycosis. *Lancet 1912* **1**: 13–15.

Sartory, A. *Les empoisonnements par les champignons* (été de 1912). Paris.

Splendore A. Zymonematosi con localizzazione nella cavità delle bocca observata in Brasile. *Bull.Soc.Path.exot.* **5**: 313–19. *Zymonema brasiliensis*

Whitfield, A. Eczematoid ringworm of the extremities and groins. *Proc. roy.Soc.Med.* **5**(1) Dermat.Sect.: 36–43. **Whitfield's ointment**

1913   Meyer, K. F. Blastomycosis in dogs. *Proc.path.Soc.Philad.* **15**: 10. **Blastomycosis (canine)**

Pinoy, E. Actinomycoses et mycétomes. *Bull.Inst. Pasteur* **11**: 929–38, 977–84.

1914   Ford, W. W. & Clark, E. D. A consideration of the properties of poisonous fungi. *Mycologia* **6**: 167–91 [60 refs].

1915–   Van Saceghem, R. Dermatose contagieuse (Impétigo conta-
16   gieux). Étude complémentaire sur la dermatose contagieuse (Impétigo contagieux). *Bull.Soc. Path.exot.* **8**: 354–9 (1915); **9**: 920–3 (1916). See also 1934. **Dermatophilosis (*Dermatophilus congolensis*)**

1916   Chalmers, A. J. & Archibald, R. G. A Soudanese maduramycosis. *Ann.trop.Med.Parasitol.* **10**: 169–222.

Naumov, N. A. *P'iany khlieb* [Intoxicating bread]. Trudy Biuro po Mik. i Fitopath. No 12. Petrograd [Leningrad]. [Reviewed *Phytopathology* **7**: 384–6 (1917).]

1918   Chalmers, A. J. & Archibald, R. G. The classification of the myceto-mas. *J.trop.Med.Hyg.* **21**: 121–3.

Giltner, L. T. The occurrence of coccidioidal granuloma (oidiomycosis) in cattle. *J.agric.Res.* **14**: 533–41. **Coccidioidomycosis (Bovine)**

1920   Smith, T. Mycosis of the bovine fetal membranes due to a mold of the genus Mucor. *J.exp.Med.* **31**: 115–22.

1920–3 Sartory, A. *Champignons parasites de l'homme et des animaux.* Paris. [Issued in 13 parts + Table des matières, and suppl.]

1921   Bloch, B. Les trichophytides. *Ann. Derm. Syph. Paris* **21**: 1–16, 55–71.

Kern, R. A. Dust sensitization in bronchial asthma. *Med. Clinics North-Am.* **5**: 751.

Neveu-Lemaire, M. *Précis de parasitologie humaine*, edn 5 [edn 1 as *Parasitologie animale* (1902).] Paris.

1922   Cooke R. A. Studies in specific hypersensitiveness. IV. New etiolo-gical factors in bronchial asthma. *J.Immunology* **7**: 147–62.

1923   Ashworth, J. H. On *Rhinosporidium seeberi* (Wernicke, 1903), with special reference to its sporulation and affinities. *Trans.roy.Soc.Edinb.* **53**: 301–38. *Rhinosporidium seeberi*

Berkhout, Christine M. *De Schimmelgeslachten Monilia, Oidium, Oospora en Torula.* Dissert. Univ. Utrecht. *Candida albicans*

Ota, M. & Langeron, M. Nouvelle classification des dermatophytes. I. Place des dermatophytes dans la classification des cryptogames. *Ann. Parasit.hum.comp.* **9**: 305–36.

Paulman, V. C. Live stock poisoning. Poisoning from burned, sweet clover hay. *Vet.Med.* **18**: 734–6.

1924   Cadman, F. T. Asthma due to grain rusts. *J.Am.med.Ass.* **83**: 27.

Sartory, A. *Guide practique des manipulations de mycologie parasitaire.* Paris.

Schofield, F. W. Damaged sweet clover: the cause of a new disease in cattle simulating hemorrhagic septicemia and blackleg. *J.Am.vet.Ass.* **64**: 553–75.

Storm van Leeuwen, W. Bronchial asthma in relation to climate. *Proc.roy. Soc.Med.* (Sect.Ther. & Pharm.) **17**: 19–26.

Witkamp, J. *Bijdrage tot de kennis van de Hyphomycosis destruens.* Thesis. Hoogeschool te Utrecht.

1925

1925   Faber, H. K. & Dickey, L. B. The treatment of thrush with gentian violet. *Am.J.Dis.Child.* **34**: 408–17.

Gilman, H. L. & Birch, R. R. A mould associated with abortion in cattle. *Cornell Vet.* **15**: 81–9.

Grigoraki, L. Recherches cytologiques et taxonomiques sur les dermatophytes et quelques autres champignons parasites. *Ann. sci.nat.Bot.*, sér. 10, **7**: 165–444.

Kingery, L. B. & Thienes, C. H. Mycotic paronychia and dermatitis: a hitherto undescribed condition apparently peculiar to fruit canners. *Arch.Derm.Syph.Chicago* **11**: 186–202. **Candidosis (paronychia)**

1926   Buxton, E. A. Mycotic vaginitis in gilts. *Vet.Med.* **22**: 451–2.

Foerster, H. R. Sporotrichosis an occupational dermatosis. *J.Am.med.Ass.* **87**: 1423–30.

1926–8 Ota, M. Champignons parasites de l'homme (Études morphologiques et systématiques). *Jap.J.Derm.Urol.* **26**: 1–28, 111–43, 751–91, 1926; **27**: 152–91, 909–38, 1927; **28**: 381–424, 1928. [Jap.; Fr. summary **28**: 18–23.]

1927   Hirsch, E. F. & Benson, H. Specific skin and testis reaction with culture filtrates of *Coccidioides immitis.* *J.infect.Dis.* **40**: 629–33.

Hirsch, E. F. & D'Andrea, D. The specific substance of *Coccidioides immitis. Ibid.* **40**: 634–7. Sensitization of guinea pigs with broth culture filtrates and with killed mycelium. *Ibid.* **40**: 638–40.

Nannizzi, A. Ricerche sull'origine saprofitica dei funghi dell tigne. Il *Gymnoascus gypseum* sp.n. forma ascofora del *Sabouraudites (Achorion) gypseum* (Bodin) Ota et Langeron. *Atti Accad.Fisiocr.Siena* **10**: 89–97.

1927–8 Castellani, A. Fungi and fungous diseases. *Arch.Derm.Syph. Chicago* **16**: 383–425, 571–604, 714–40 (1927); **17**: 61–97, 194–220, 354–79 (1928). [Reprinted as a book, 1928, Chicago.]

1928   Alexander, A. *et al. Dermatomykosen.* Berlin. [= J. Jadassohn, *Handbuch der Haut- und Geschlechtskrankheiten*, Band 11.]

Bloch, B. Allgemeine und experimentelle Biologie der durch Hyphomyceten erzeugten Dermatomykosen. In Alexander *et al.* (1928): 300–77; Die Trichophytide, *Ibid.*: 565–606.

Castellani, A. The treatment of epidermophytosis of the toes (mango toe) and certain forms of epidermophytosis by fuchsin paint. *Lancet 1928* **2**: 595–6. **Castellani's paint**

Cavara, V. *Le micosi oculari.* Siena. [= *Trattato di Mycopathologia Umana*, **3**.]

Connor, C. L. *Monilia* from osteomyelitis. *J.infect.Dis.* **43**: 108–16. **Candidosis (osteomyelitis)**

Fonseca, O. da & Arêa Leão, A. C. Sobre os cogumelos da piedra Brasileira. *Mem.Inst.Oswaldo Cruz. Suppl.das Mem.* 4 des de 1928: 124–7. *Piedraia hortai*

Guiart, J. & Grigorakis, L. La classification botanique des champignons des teignes. *Lyon Médical* **141**: 369–78.

Robertson, J. & Ashby, H. T. Ergot poisoning among rye bread consumers. *Br.med.J. 1928* **1**: 302–3.

1928-9   Ravaut, P. & Rabeau, H. Parakératoses psoriasiformes sèches et levûrides. *Presse Méd.* **36**: 1443–6, 1928; Parakératoses eczemati-formes provoquées par des injections intradermiques de levûrine; *ibid.* **37**: 372–5 (1929).

1929   Bendixen, H. C. & Plum, N. Schimmelpilze (*Aspergillus fumigatus* und *Absidia ramosa*) als Abortusursache beim Rinde. *Acta path.microbiol. Scand.* **6**: 252–322. **Bovine mycotic abortion**

Frost, K., Sutherland-Campbell, H. & Plunkett, O. A. Monilia of the tongue. Report of an incidence with associated skin lesions. *Arch.Derm. Syph. Chicago* **20**: 811–19.

*Garrison, F. H. *An introduction to the history of medicine*, edn 4. Philadelphia & London.

Grigorakis, L. Dermatophytes and dermatomycoses. *Ann. Derm.Syph.Paris* sér. 6, **10**: 18–68.

Margarot, T. & Devèze, P. La lumière de Wood en dermatologie. *Ann.Derm. Syph.Paris* sér. 6, **10**: 581–608. **Wood's light**

Morgan, M. T. Report on an outbreak of alleged ergot poisoning by rye bread in Manchester. *J.Hygiene* **29**: 51–61.

Sabouraud, R. Généralités concernant les dermatophytes. 6e mémoire. De la classification naturelle des dermatophytes. *Ann.Derm.Syph.Paris* sér. 6,**10**: 569–80.

1930   de Almeida, F. Estudos comparativos do granuloma coccidioidico nos Estados Unidos e no Brasil. Novo genero para o parasito brasileiro. *Annais Fac.Med.Univ.S.Paulo* **5**: 3–19. *Paracoccidioides brasiliensis*

Bernton, H. S. Asthma due to a mold, *Aspergillus fumigatus. J.Am.med.Ass.* **95**: 189.

Henrici, A. T. *Molds, yeasts and actinomycetes*. New York. [edn 2, by C. E. Skinner, C. W. Emmons & H. M. Tsuchiya (1947).]

Hopkins, J. G., Benham, Rhoda W. & Kesten, B. M. Asthma due to a fungus, Alternaria. *J.Am.med.Ass.* **94**: 6.

Langeron, M. & Milochevitch, S. Morphologie des dermatophytes sur les milieux naturels et milieux á base de polysaccharides. *Ann.Parasit. hum.comp.* **8**: 422–6, 465–508.

1931   Barger, G. *Ergot and ergotism*. London & Edinburgh.

Benham, Rhoda W. Certain monilias parasitic on man; their identification by morphology and by agglutination. *J.infect.Dis.* **49**: 183–215.

Kinnear, J. Wood's glass in the diagnosis of ringworm. *Br.med.J. 1931* **1**: 791–3.

Lôbo, J. Chromoblastomycoses. *Revta med.Permanb.* 1: 763–6.
Lobomycosis

Lundquist, C. W. On primary mycosis of the kidney. *Br.J.Urol* 3: 1–13.
Candidosis (nephritis)

Redaelli, P. *Tecnica micologica medica.* Bologna.

Vuillemin, P. *Les champignons parasites et les mycoses de l'homme.* Paris.

1932   Benham, Rhoda W. & Kesten, B. Sporotrichosis: its transmission to plants and animals. *J.infect.Dis.* 50: 437–58.

Campbell, J. M. Acute symptoms following work with hay. *Br.med.J.* *1932* 2: 1143–4.

Cobe, H. M. Asthma due to a mold *Cladosporium fulvum*. *J.Allergy* 3: 389.

Jacobson, H. P. *Fungus diseases: a clinico-mycological text.* Springfield, Ill.

Kanouse, Bessie B. A physiological and morphological study of *Saprolegnia parasitica*. *Mycologia* 24: 431–52.

Langeron, M. & Talice, R. V. Nouvelles méthodes d'étude et essai de classification des champignons levuriformes. *Ann.Parasit.hum.comp.* 10: 1–80.

Stewart, R. A. & Meyer, K. F. Isolation of *Coccidioides immitis* (Stiles) from the soil. *Proc.Soc.exp.Biol.Med.* 29: 937–8.

Towey, J. W., Sweaney, H. C. & Huron, W. H. Severe bronchial asthma apparently due to fungus spores found in maple bark. *J.Am.med.Ass.* 99: 453–9.

1933   Catanei, A. Études sur les teignes. *Arch.Inst.Pasteur Alger.* 11: 267–399.

Davidson, A. M. & Gregory, P. H. Development of fuseaux, aleurispores, and spirals on detached hairs infected by ringworm fungi. *Nature* 131: 836–7. [See also 1934.]

Steyn, D. G. Fungi in relation to health in man and animals. *Onderspoort J.vet.Sci.animal Industr.* 1: 183–212.

1934   Benham, Rhoda W. Fungi of blastomycosis and coccidioidal granuloma. *Arch.Derm.Syph.Chicago* 30: 385–400.

Davidson, A. M. & Gregory, P. H. *In situ* cultures of dermatophytes. *Can.J.Res.* 10: 373–93. [See also 1933.]

DeMonbreun, W. A. The cultivation and cultural characteristics of Darling's *Histoplasma capsulatum*. *Am.J.trop.Med.* 14: 93–126.

Dodd, Katherine & Tomkins, E. H. A case of histoplasmosis of Darling in an infant. *Am.J.trop.Med.* 14: 127–37.

Emmons, C. W. Dermatophytes. Natural grouping based on the form of the spores and accessory organs. *Arch.Derm.Syph.Chicago* 30: 337–62.

Hansmann, G. H. & Schenken, J. R. A unique infection in man caused by a new yeast-like organism, a pathogenic member of the genus *Sepedonium*. *Am.J.Path.* 10: 731–8.

Nannizzi, A. *Repertio sistematico dei miceti dell'uomo e degli animali.* Siena. [= *Trattato di micopatologia umana* 4.]

Van Saceghem, R. La dermatose, dit contagieuse des bovides. Impetigo tropical des bovides. *Bull.agric.Congo belge* **25**: 590–8 (See also 1915–16.)

1935　Dodge, C. W. *Medical mycology.* St Louis, Mo. & London.

Feinberg, S. M. Mold allergy: its importance in asthma and hay fever. *Wisconsin med.J.* **34**: 254.

Gomez–Vega, Paulina. Mycostatic studies on certain moniliae and related fungi. *Arch.Derm.Syph.Chicago* **32**: 49–58.

de Magalhães, O. Ensaios de micologia. *Mem.Inst. Oswaldo Cruz* **30**: 1–55.

1936　Brown, G. T. Hypersensitivity to fungi. *J.Allergy* **7**: 455–70.

Gordon, R. E. & Hagan, W. A. A study of some acid-fast actinomycetes from soil with special reference to pathogenicity for animals. *J.infect. Dis.* **59**: 200–6.

Hopkirk, C. S. M. Paspalum staggers. *N.Z.J.Agric.* **53**: 105–8.

Shrewsbury, J. F. D. Secondary thrush of the bronchi. *Quart.J.med.* **29** [NS 5]: 375–97.

1936–7　Conant, N. F. *Studies on the genus Microsporum.* I. Cultural studies [1936]; II. Biometric studies [1936]; III. Taxonomic studies [1937]. *Arch.Derm. Syph.Chicago* **33**: 665–83; **34**: 79–89, 1936; **35**: 781–808 (1937).

1937　Castellani, A. A short general account for medical men of the genus *Monilia*, Persoon, 1797. *J.trop.Med.Hyg.* **40**: 293–307.

Conant N. F. The occurrence of a human pathogenic fungus as a saprophyte in nature. *Mycologia* **29**: 597–8.

Dickson, E. C. *Coccidioides* infection I. *Arch.intl.Med.* **57**: 1029–44.

Mandlick, G. S. A record of rhinosporidial polypi with some observations on the mode of infection. *Indian med.Gaz.* **72**: 143–7.

Muende, I. & Webb, P. Ringworm fungus growing as a saprophyte under natural conditions. *Arch.Derm.Syph.Chicago* **36**: 987–90.

1938　*Bulloch, W. *The history of bacteriology.* Oxford. [Reprinted, 1960.]

Cope, Z. *Actinomycosis.* London.

Dévé, F. Une nouvelle forme anatomo-radiologique de mycose pulmonaire primitive. Le méga-mycétome intra-bronchectasique. *Arch.Med.Chir. appl.Resp.* **5**: 337–61. **Aspergilloma**

Dickson, E. C. & Gifford, Myrnie A. *Coccidioides* infection (coccidioido-mycosis). II. The primary type of infection. *Arch.intl.Med.* **62**: 853–71.

Dujarric de la Rivière, R. & Heim, R. *Les champignons toxiques.* Paris. [600 refs.]

Durham, O. C. An unusual shower of fungal spores. *J.Am.med.Ass.* **111**: 24–5.

Emmons, C. W. The isolation of *Actinomyces bovis* from tonsillar granules. *Publ.Health Rep.Wash.* **53**: 1967–75.

Rao, M. Anant Narayan. Rhinosporidiosis in bovines in the Madras Presidency, with a discussion on the probable modes of infection. *Indian J.vet.Sci.* **8**: 187–98.

1939　Almeida, F. P. de. *Mycologia medica.* São Paulo.

Benham, Rhoda, W. The cultural characteristics of *Pityrosporum ovale* – a lipophylic fungus. *J.invest.Derm* **2**: 187–202.

Conant, N. F. Laboratory study of *Blastomyces dermatitidis* Gilchrist & Stokes 1898. *Sixth Pacific Sci. Conf.* **5**: 853–62.

DeMonbreun, W. A. & Anderson, K. The dog as a natural host for *Histoplasma capsulatum*. Report of a case of histoplasmosis in this animal. *Am.J.trop.Med.* **19**: 565–87. **Histoplasmosis (canine)**

Kirschenblatt, J. D. A new parasite of the lungs of rodents. *CR(Doklady) Acad.Sci URSS* **23**: 406–8. **Adiaspiromycosis**

Knighton, H. T. A study of Monilia and other yeastlike organisms found in the oral cavity. *J.dent.Res.* **18**: 103–25.

Lewis, G. M. & Hopper, Mary E. *An introduction to medical mycology.* Chicago. [edn 4, 1958.]

Negroni, P. Reseña histórica de la micología médica argentina. *Mycopathologia* **1**: 267–70. [Suppl. *ibid.* **8**: 216–38 (1957).]

Oxford, A. E., Raistrick, H. & Simonart, P. Studies in the biochemistry of micro-organisms. 60. Griseofulvin, a metabolic product of *Penicillium griseofulvum* Dierckx. *Biochem.J.* **33**: 240–8.

Tiffney, W. N. The host range of *Saprolegnia parasitica. Mycologia* **31**: 310–21.

1940   *Emmons, C. W. Medical mycology. *Bot.Rev.* **6**: 474–514. [311 refs.]

Fonseca, O. da & Arêa Leão, A. E. de. Contribuição para o conhecimento das granulumatoses blastomicoides. O agente etiologico da micose de Jorge Lobo. *Rev.Med.Cir.Brasil* **48**: 147–58. *Glenosporella loboi*

Joachim, H. & Polayes, S. H. Subacute endocarditis and systemic mycosis (*Monilia*). *J.Am.med.Ass.* **115**: 205–8. **Candidosis (endocarditis)**

Miyake, I., Naito, H. & Tsunoda, H. Study of toxin production of stored rice by parasitic fungi. *Rep.Rice Utilization Res.Inst.,Min.Agric.Forestry* **1**.

1941   Conant, N. F. A cultural study of the life-cycle of *Histoplasma capsulatum* Darling 1906. *J.Bact.* **41**: 563–80.

Gastineau, F. M., Spolyar, L. W. & Haynes, Edith. Sporotrichosis. Report of six cases among florists. *J.Am.med.Ass.* **117**: 1074–7.

Raistrick, H. & Smith, G. Antibacterial substances from moulds. I. Citrinin, a metabolic product of *Penicillium citrinum* Thom. *Chem.Ind.* **60**: 828–30.

Curasson, G. *Traité de pathologie exotique vétérinaire et comparée. 2. Maladies microbiennes.* Paris. [Epizootic lymphangitis, pp. 205–57.]

1942   Davis, B. L., Smith, Ruth T. & Smith, C. E. An epidemic of coccidioidal infection (coccidioidomycosis). *J.Am.med.Ass.* **118**: 1182–6.

Emmons, C. W. Isolation of Coccidioides from soil and rodents. *Publ.Health Rep.Wash.* **57**: 109–11.

Emmons, C. W. & Ashburn, L. L. The isolation of *Haplosporangium parvum* n.sp. and *Coccidioides immitis* from wild rodents. Their relationship to coccidioidomycosis. *Publ.Health Rep.Wash.* **57**: 1715–27.

Negroni, P. *Dermatomicosis. Diagnostico y tratamiento.* Buenos Aires.

Redaelli, P. & Ciferri, R. *Le granulomatosi fungine dell'uomo nelle regioni tropicali e subtropicali.* Florence. [= *Trattata di micopatologia umana* **5**.]

1943   Morrow, Marie B. & Lowe, E. P. Molds in relation to asthma and vasomotor rhinitis. *Mycologia* **35**: 638–53.

Redaelli, P. & Ciferri, R. Relazione sul primo quinquennio (1938–43) di attività del Centro di Micologia Umana e Comparatava della R.Università di Pavia. *Atti Ist.bot. Univ.Lab.crittogam. Pavia* sér. 5, **3**: 1–90.

Smith, C. E. Coccidioidomycosis. *Med.Clin.N.Am.* **27**: 790–808.

1944   Conant, N. F., Martin, D. S., Smith, D. T., Baker, R. D. & Callaway, J. L. *Manual of clinical mycology*. Philadelphia. [edn 3 (1971).]

Duché, J. À propos du 'mal des cannes de Provence'. *Rec.Trav.Inst.Nat. Hyg.Paris* **2**: 242–52.

Emmons, C. W. *Allescheria boydii* and *Monosporium apiospermum*. *Mycologia* **36**: 188–93. ***Allescheria boydii***

Negroni, P. & Fischer, Ida. *Pseudallescheria sheari* n.gen., n.sp. aislada de un para micetoma de la rodilla. *Rev.Inst.bact.B.Aires* **12**: 195–204. ***Pseudallescheria***

*Zakon, S. J. & Benedek, T. David Gruby and the centenary of medical mycology, 1841–1941. *Bull.Hist.Med.* **16**: 155–68. [Engl.transl. of Gruby's 6 papers to the French Academy.]

1945   Christie, A. & Peterson, J. C. Pulmonary calcification in negative reaction to tuberculin. *Am.J.publ.Health* **35**: 1131–47.

Duncan, J. T. A survey of fungus diseases in Great Britain. Results from the first 18 months. *Br.med.J.* 1945 **2**: 715–18.

Emmons, C. W. & Hollaender, A. Relation of ultraviolet induced mutations to speciation in dermatophytes. *Arch.Derm. Syph.Chicago* **52**: 257–61.

Hyde, H. A. & Williams, D. A. Studies in atmospheric pollen II. Diurnal variation in incidence of grass pollen. *New.Phytol.* **44**: 83–94.

Langeron, M. *Précis de mycologie*. Paris. [edn 2, by R. Vanbreuseghem (1952).]

Palmer, C. E. Nontuberculous pulmonary calcification and sensitivity to histoplasmin. *Pub.Health Rep.Wash.* **60**: 513–20.

Parsons, R. J. & Zarafonetis, C. Histoplasmosis in man: report of seven cases and a review of seventy-one cases. *Arch.intern.Med.* **75**: 1–23.

1946   Brian, P. W., Curtis, P. J. & Hemming, H. G. A substance causing abnormal development of fungal hyphae produced by *Penicillium janczewskii* Zal. I. Biological assay, production and isolation of 'curling factor'. *Trans. Br.mycol.Soc.* **29**: 173–87.

Cox, L. B. & Tolhurst, Jean C. *Human torulosis. A clinical, pathological and microbiological study and a report of thirteen cases*. Melbourne Univ. Press.

Gomori, G. A new histochemical test for glycogen and mucin. *Am.J. clin.Path.* **10** (Tech.Bull.Registry med.Technologists 7): 177–9.

Levine, S. & Ordal, Z. J. Factors influencing the morphology of *Blastomyces dermatitidis*. *J.Bact.* **52**: 687–94.

Smith, C. E., Beard, R. R., Rosenberger, H. G. & Whiting, E. G. Effect of season and dust control on coccidioidomycosis. *J.Am.med.Ass.* **132**: 833–8.

1947   Campbell, Charlotte C. Reverting *Histoplasma capsulatum* to the yeast phase. *J.Bact.* **54**: 263–4.

Feinberg, S. M. *Allergy in practice.* Chicago. [Allergy to fungi pp. 216–84, 136 refs.]

Grove, J. F. & McGowen, J. C. Identity of griseofulvin and 'curling factor'. *Nature* **160**: 574.

Hazen, Elizabeth L. *Microsporum audouinii*: the effect of yeast extract, thiamine, pyridoxine, and *Bacillus weidmaniensis* on the colony characteristics and micro-conidial formation. *Mycologia* **39**: 200–9.

Hirata, Y. On the products of a mould. I. Poisonous substances from mouldy rice. (Part I) Extraction. *J.chem.Soc.Japan* **65**: 63.

Keddie, J. A. G. Ringworm of the scalp in children. Its causation, detection, and treatment, and a report on an outbreak. *Health Bull.* (Dept Health Scotl.) **5**: 66–8.

Leach, B. E., Ford, J. H. & Whiffen, Alma J. Actidione, an antibiotic from *Streptomyces griseus.* *J.Am.chem.Soc.* **69**: 474. **Actidione**

Nickerson, W. J. (ed). *Biology of pathogenic fungi.* Waltham, Mass.

Rewell, R. E. & Ainsworth, G. C. Occurrence of *Aspergillus fumigatus* in the lung of an American bison. *Nature* **160**: 362–3.

Rothman, S., Smiljanic, Adelaide M., Shapiro, A. L. & Weitkamp, A. W. The spontaneous cure of tinea capitis in puberty. *J.invest.Derm.* **8**: 81–98.

Skinner, C. E. The yeast-like fungi: *Candida* and *Brettanomyces. Bact Rev.* **11**: 227–74. (303 refs). [Suppl. *ibid.* **24**: 397–416 (1960) 227 refs.]

Smith, D. T. *Fungus diseases of the lungs.* Springfield, Ill. [edn 2 (1963).]

Sporotrichosis infection in mines of the Witwatersrand. A symposium. Johannesburg (Transvaal Chamber of Mines).

1947–   Duncan, J. T. A unique form of *Histoplasma. Trans.R.Soc.trop.*
58   *Med.Hyg.* **40**: 364–5 (1947): Tropical African histoplasmosis. *Ibid.* **52**: 468–74, 1958.

1948   Benbrook, E. A., Bryant, J. B. & Saunders, L. Z. A case of blastomycosis in the horse. *J.Am.vet.med.Ass.* **112**: 475–8. **Blastomycosis (equine)**

Benham, Rhoda W. Effect of nutrition on growth and morphology of the dermatophytes. I. Development of microconidia in *Trichophyton rubrum. Mycologia* **40**: 232–40.

Mackinnon, J. E. Las condiciones meteorológicas causa determinante de la frequencia de la esporotricosis. *Ann.Inst.Hig.Montevideo* **2**: 50–68.

Mackinnon, J. E. & Artagaveytia-Allende, R. C. Diferentes 'auxoheterotrofias' en cepas de hongos de la misma especie. *Ann.Inst.Hig.Montevideo* **2** :11–31.

Nichols, D. R. & Herrell, W. E. Penicillin in the treatment of actinomycosis. *J.lab.clin.Med.* **33**: 521–5.

Prchal, C. J. Coccidioidomycosis of cattle in Arizona. *J.Am.vet.med.Ass.* **112**: 461–3.

Richman, H. Histoplasmosis in a colt. *N.Am.Vet.* **29**: 170. **Histoplasmosis (equine)**

1949   Bullen, J. J. The yeast-like form of *Cryptococcus farciminosus* (*Histoplasma farciminosum*). *J.Path.Bact.* **61**: 117–20.

Emmons, C. W. Isolation of *Histoplasma capsulatum* from soil. *Publ.Health Rep.Wash.* **64**: 892–6.

Furcolow, M. L. & Ruhe, J. S. Histoplasma sensitivity among cattle. *Am.J.publ.Health* **39**: 719–21.

Georg, Lucille. Influence of nutrition on growth and morphology of dermatophytes. *Trans.N.Y.Acad.Sci.* ser. 2, **11**: 281–6.

Mackinnon, J. E. The dependence on the weather of the incidence of sporotrichosis. *Mycopathologia* **4**: 367–74.

Salvin, S. B. Phase-determining factors in *Blastomyces dermatitidis*. *Mycologia* **41**: 311–19.

Vanbreuseghem, R. La culture des dermatophytes *in vitro* sur des cheveux isolés. *Ann.Parasit.hum.comp.* **24**: 559–73. [See also *Mycologia* **44**: 176–82 (1952).]

1950

1950   Akün, R. S. Histoplasmosis in a cat. *J.Am.vet.med.Ass.* **117**: 43–4. **Histoplasmosis (feline)**

Blaxland, J. D. & Fincham, I. H. Mycosis of the crop (moniliasis) in poultry. With particular reference to serious mortality in young turkeys. *Br.vet.J.* **106**: 221–31. **Candidosis (avian)**

*Carneiro, A. L. Ten years investigation about mycopathology in Portugal (1938–1948). *Mycopathologia* **5**: 91–4.

Emmons, C. W. The natural occurrence in animals and soil of fungi which cause disease in man. *Proc.Seventh internat.bot Congr.Stockholm*: 416–21.

Georg, Lucille. The relation of nutrition to the growth and morphology of *Trichophyton faviforme*. *Mycologia* **42**: 693–716.

Iams, A. M. Histoplasmin skin test. *Ann.N.Y.Acad.Sci.* **50**: 1380–7.

Kligman, A. M. & Mescon, H. The periodic-acid-Schiff stain for the demonstration of fungi in animal tissue. *J.Bact.* **60**: 415–21.

*Niño, F. L. Hallazgo de una pieza anatomica; su importancia en la historia de la Psorospermiosis o granulada coccidioidico. *Bol.Inst. clin.quir.* **26**: 3–14.

Peck, S. M. Fungus antigens and their importance as sensitizers in the general population. *Ann.N.Y.Acad.Sci.* **50**: 1362–75.

1951 *Ainsworth, G. C. A century of medical and veterinary mycology in Britain. *Trans.Br.mycol.Soc.* **34**: 1–16.

Ajello, L. & Zeidberg, L. D. Isolation of *Histoplasma capsulatum* and *Allescheria boydii* from soil. *Science* **113**: 662–3.

Emmons, C. W. Isolation of *Cryptococcus neoformans* from soil. *J.Bact.* **62**: 685–90.

Frankland, A. W. & Hay, M. J. Dry rot as a cause of allergic complaints. *Acta Allergololica* **4**: 186–200.

*Gray, Sir A. Dermatology from the time of Harvey. *Lancet 1951* **2**: 795.

Gregory, P. H. Deposition of air-borne *Lycopodium* spores on cylinders. *Ann.appl.Biol.* **38**: 357–76.

Hazen, Elizabeth L. & Brown, Rachael. Fungicidin [**Nystatin**], an antibiotic produced by a soil actinomycete. *Proc.Soc.exp.Biol.N.Y.* **76**: 93–7.

1952 Ainsworth, G. C. *Medical mycology. An introduction to its problems.* London (Pitmans).

*Backman, E. L. *Religious dances in the Christian church and popular medicine.* London.

Drouhet, E. & Mariat, F. Étude des facteurs determinant le développement de la phase levure de *Sporotrichum schencki*. *Ann.Inst.Pasteur* **83**: 506–14.

Dubois, A., Janssens, P. G. & Brutsaert, P. Un cas d'histoplasmose africaine. Avec une note mycologique sur *Histoplasma duboisii* n.sp. par R. Vanbreuseghem. *Ann.Soc.belg.Med.trop.* **32**: 569–83.

Georg, Lucille. Cultural and nutritional studies of *Trichophyton gallinae* and *Trichophyton megninii*. *Mycologia* **44**: 470–92.

Gregory, P. H. Spore content of the atmosphere near the ground. *Nature.* **170**: 475–7.

Hirst, J. An automatic volumetric spore trap. *Ann.appl.Biol.* **39**: 257–65.

Kligman, A. M. The pathogenesis of tinea capitis due to *Microsporum audouini* and *Microsporum canis*. I. Gross observations following the inoculation of humans. *J.invest.Derm.* **18**:231–45.

La Touche, C. J. The Leeds campaign against microsporosis in children and domestic animals. *Vet.Rec.* **64**: 398–9.

Lodder, Jacomina & Krieger-van Rij, Nellie J. W. *The yeasts – a taxonomic study.* Amsterdam. [edn. 3 (1984) (Krieger-van Rij, ed.).]

McErlean, B. A. Vulvovaginitis in swine. *Vet.Rec.* **64**: 539–40.

Nickerson, W. J. Report of a Committee on medical and veterinary mycology [of the International Congress of Microbiology]. *Internat. Bull.bact.Nomen.Tax.* **2**: 143–50.

Silva, Margarita & Benham, Rhoda W. Nutrition studies of the dermatophytes with special reference to *Trichophyton megnini* Blanchard 1896 and *Trichophyton gallinae* (Megnin 1981) comb.nov. *J.invest.Derm.* **18**: 453–72.

Vanbreuseghem, R. Technique biologique pour l'isolement des dermatophytes du sol. *Ann.Soc.belg.Méd.trop.* **32**: 173–8.

Zeidberg, L. D., Ajello, L., Dillon, Ann & Runyon, Laliah C. Isolation of *Histoplasma capsulatum* from soil. *Am.J.publ.Health* **42**: 930–5.

1953   Benham, Rhoda W. Nutritional studies of the dermatophytes. Effect on growth and morphology, with special reference to the production of macroconidia. *Trans.N.Y.Acad.Sci.* ser. 2, **15**: 102–6.

Durie, E. Beatrix & Brown, Shirley. Fungus infections in hospital practice. *Med.J.Australia* **40**: 813–14.

Fuller, C. J. Farmer's lung: a review of present knowledge. *Thorax* **8**: 59–64.

Grayston, T. J. & Furcolow, M. L. The occurrence of histoplasmosis in epidemics – epidemiological studies. *Am.J.publ.Health* **43**: 665–76; – etiologic studies. *Am.Rev.Tuberc.* **68**: 307–20.

Gridley, Mary. F. A stain for fungi in tissue sections. *Am.Rev.clin.Path.* **23**: 303–7.

*Mayer, C. F. Endemic panmyelotoxicosis in the Russian Grain Belt. Part one: The clinical aspects of alimentary toxic aleukia (ATA). A comprehensive review. *Mil.Surg.* **113**: 173–89. Part two: The botany, phytopathology, and toxicology of Russian cereal food. *Ibid.* **113**: 295–315.

Moss, Emma S. & McQuown, A. L. *Atlas of medical mycology.* Baltimore. [edn 3 (1969).]

Nickerson, W. J. & Mankowski, Z. Role of nutrition in the maintenance of the yeast-shape in *Candida. Am.J.Bot.* **40**: 584–92.

1954   Georg, Lucille K., Ajello, L. & Papageorge, Calomira. Use of cyclohexamide in the selective isolation of fungi pathogenic to man. *J.lab.clin.Med.* **44**: 422–8.

*Kisch, B. Forgotten leaders in modern medicine. Valentin, Gruby, Remak, Auerbach. *Trans.Am.phil.Soc.* NS **44**: 139–316.

Menges, R. W. Histoplasmin sensitivity in animals. *Cornell Vet.* **44**: 21–31.

Negroni, P. *Micosis profundis (cutaneas y viscerales).* I. *Los micetomas.* Buenos Aires.

Sarkisov, A. K. [*Mycotoxicoses (Fungus poisons)*]. Moscow. [Russ.]

1955   Ainsworth, G. C. & Austwick, P. K. C. A survey of animal mycoses in Britain. General aspects. *Vet.Rec.* **67**: 88–97; Mycological aspects. *Trans.Br. mycol.Soc.* **38**: 369–86.

Converse, J. L. Growth of spherules of *Coccidioides immitis* in a chemically defined liquid medium. *Proc.Soc.exp.Biol. N.Y.* **90**: 709–11.

Di Menna, Margaret E. A search for pathogenic species of yeasts in New Zealand soils. *J.gen.Microbiol.* **12**: 54–62.

Emmons, C. W. Saprophytic sources of *Cryptococcus neoformans* associated with the pigeon (*Columba livia*). *Am.J.Hyg.* **62**: 227–32.

Grocott, R. C. A stain for fungi in tissue and smears using Gomori's methenamine-silver nitrate technic. *Am.J.clin.Path.* **25**: 975–9.

Hazen, Elizabeth C. & Reed, F. C. *Laboratory identification of pathogenic fungi simplified.* Oxford. [edn 2 (1960).]

Kligman, A. M. Tinea capitis due to *M. audouini* and *M. canis.* II. Dynamics of the host-parasite relationship. *Arch. Derm.Syph. Chicago* **71**: 313–37.

La Touche, C. J. The importance of the animal reservoir of infection in the epidemiology of animal-type ringworm in man. *Vet.Rec.* **57**: 666–7.

Lurie, H. I. Fungal diseases in South Africa. *S.Afr.med.J.* **29**: 186–8.

Stuart, E. A. & Blank, F. Aspergillosis of the ear. A report of twenty-nine cases. *Can.med.Ass.J.* **72** 334–7.

Vanbreuseghem, R. Le Congo Belge et la mycologie médicale. *Acad.roy.Sci.col., Class Sci.nat.med. Mem.in 8° NS 1(1).* [Brussels.]

1956   Abbott, P. Mycetoma in the Sudan. *Trans.R.Soc.trop.Med.Hyg.* **50**: 11–30.

Feller, A. E., Furcolow, M. L., Larsh, H. W., Langmuir, A. D. & Dingle, J. H. Outbreak of unusual form of pneumonia at Camp Gruber, Oklahoma, in 1944. *Am.J.Med.* **21**: 184–92.

Gentles, J. C. The isolation of dermatophytes from floors of communal bathing places. *J.clin.Path.* **9**: 374–7.

Gold, W., Stout, H. A., Pagano, J. F. & Donovick, R. Amphotericins A and B, antifungal antibiotics produced by a streptomycete. I. *In vitro* studies. *Antibiotics Annual 1955–56*: 579–86. **Amphotericin B**

Joe, L. K., Eng, N.-I. T., Van der Meulen, H. & Emmons, C. W. *Basidiobolus ranarum* as a cause of subcutaneous mycosis in Indonesia. *Arch.Derm.Syph.Chicago* **75**: 378–83. **Phycomycosis (*Basidiobolus ranarum*)**

Kligman, A. M. Pathophysiology of ringworm infections in animals with skin cycles. *J.invest.Derm.* **27**: 171–85.

Koelle, W. A. & Pastor, B. H. *Candida albicans* endocarditis after aortic valvulotomy. *New.Engl.J.Med.* **225**: 997–8.

Littman, M. L. & Zimmerman, L. E. *Cryptococcosis.* New York.

Marples, Mary J. The ecology of *Microsporum canis* in New Zealand. *J.Hyg.* **54**: 378–87.

Smith, C. E., Saito, Margaret T. & Simons, Susan A. Pattern of 39,5000 serologic tests in coccidioidomycosis. *J.Am.med.Ass.* **160**: 546–52.

Zapater, R. C. *Atlas de diagnóstica micológica de laboratorio.* Buenos Aires. [edn 3 (1973).]

1957   Ajello, L. The Communicable Disease Center's film teaching aids in medical mycology. *Trans.N.Y.Acad.Sci.* **20**: 75–8.

Beneke, E. S. *Medical mycology. Laboratory manual.* Minneapolis.

Bridges, C. H. Maduromycotic mycetomas in animals. *Curvularia geniculata* as an etiologic agent. *Am.J.Path.* **33**: 411–27.

Burnside, J. E., Sippel, W. L., Forgacs, J., Carll, W. T., Atwood, M. B. & Doll, E. R. A disease of swine and cattle caused by eating moldy corn II. Experimental production with pure cultures of molds. *Am.J.vet.Res.* **18**: 817–24.

Drouhet, E. Quelques aspects biologiques et mycologiques de i'histoplasmoses. *Path.Biol. Paris* **33**: 439–61.

Gentles, J. C. & Holmes, J. G. Foot ringworm in coal-mines. *Br.J.industr.Med.* **14**: 22–9.

Lie-Kian-Joe, Tjoei Eng, N. I. & Kertopati, S. A new verrucous mycosis caused by *Cercospora apii. Arch.Derm.Syph.Chicago* 75: 864–70. [See also *Mycologia* 49: 1–10, 773–4 (1957).]

*Smithcors, J. F. *Evolution of the veterinary art. A narrative account to 1850.* London.

*Wasson, V. P. & R. G. *Mushrooms, Russia and History*, 2 vols. New York.

1958   *Campins, H. Sintesis de las investigaciones micologicas realizadas en Venezuela durante los anos 1946 – 1956. *Mycopathologia* 9: 152–75.

*Ciferri, R. & Redaelli, P. *Bibliographica mycopathologica (1800–1940)*, 2 vols. [14,506 refs.] Florence (= *Biblioteca Bibliografica Italica* 18, 20.)

Emmons, C. W. Association of bats with histoplasmosis. *Publ.Health Rep.Wash.* 73: 590–5.

Fiese, M. J. *Coccidioidomycosis.* Springfield, Ill. [968 refs. History pp. 10–22.]

Furcolow, M. L. Recent studies on the epidemiology of histoplasmosis. *Ann.N.Y.Acad.Sci.* 72: 127–64.

Gentles, J. C. Experimental ringworm in guinea pigs: oral treatment with griseofulvin. *Nature* 182: 476–7. **Griseofulvin**

Heim, R. & Wasson, R. G. *et al. Les champignons hallucinogènes du Mexique.* Paris (Mus.Nat.Hist.Natur.).

Lauder, I. M. & O'Sullivan, J. G. Ringworm in cattle. Prevention and treatment with griseofulvin. *Vet.Rec.* 70: 949–51.

Percival, J. C. & Thornton, R. H. Relationship between the presence of fungal spores and a test for hepatotoxic grass. *Nature* 182: 1095–6. **Facial eczema**

Pine, L. & Peacock, C. L. Studies on the growth of *Histoplasma capsulatum.* IV. Factors influencing the conversion of the mycelial to the yeast phase. *J.Bact.* 75: 167–74.

Riddel, R. W. & Clayton, Yvonne M. Pulmonary mycoses occurring in Britain. *Br.J.Tuberc.* 52: 34–44.

Singer, R. Mycological investigations on teonanácatl, the Mexican hallucinogenic mushroom. Part I. *Mycologia* 50: 239–61. Part II (with A. H. Smith). *Ibid.* 50: 262–303.

Van der Werff, P. J. *Mould fungi and bronchial asthma. A mycological and clinical study*, vol. 1 [no more published]. Leiden. [500+ refs.]

Van Uden, N., Do Carmo Sousa, Lidia & Farinha, Manuela. On the intestinal flora of horses, sheep, goats and swine. *J.gen.Microbiol.* 19: 435–45.

Williams, D. I., Marten, R. H. & Sarkany, I. Oral treatment of ringworm with griseofulvin. *Lancet 1958* 2: 259–66.

1959   Ainsworth, G. C. & Austwick, P. K. C. *Fungal diseases of animals.* Farnham Royal (Commonw.Agric. Bur.). [edn 2 (1973).]

Ciferri, R. & Montemartini, A. The taxonomy of *Haplosporangium parvum. Mycopathologia* 10: 303–16.

Dawson, Christine O. & Gentles, J. C. Perfect state of *Keratomyces ajelloi. Nature,* 183: 1345–6.

English, Mary P. & Gibson, Mary D. Studies in the epidemiology of tinea pedis. I. Tinea pedis in school children. II. Dermatophytes on the floors of swimming baths. *Br.med.J.* 1959 1: 1442–6; 1446–8.

Kaplan, W. (a) The occurrence of black piedra in primate pelts. *Trop. geogr.Med.* 11: 115–26. (b) Piedra in lower animals. A case report of white piedra in a monkey and a review of the literature. *J.Am.vet. med.Ass.* 134: 113–17.

*Kashkin, P. N. Review of works on medical mycology published in the U.S.S.R. between 1946–1956. *Mycopathologia* 10: 227–68.

O'Dell, B. L., Regan, W. O. & Beach, T. J. A study of the toxic principle in red clover. *Miss.Univ.Agric.Exp.Stn Res.Bull.* 702.

Thornton, R. H. & Percival, J. C. A hepatotoxin from *Sporodesmium bakeri* capable of producing facial eczema disease in sheep. *Nature* 183: 63.

1960   Ajello, L. Geographic distribution and prevalence of dermatophytes. *Ann.N.Y.Acad.Sci.* 89: 20–38.

Bilaï, V. I. (ed.) *Mycotoxicoses of man and agricultural animals.* Kiev.

Bridges, C. H. Maduromycosis of bovine nasal mucosa (nasal granuloma of cattle). *Cornell Vet.* 50: 468–84.

Bridges, C. H. & Beasley, J. N. Maduromycotic mycetomas in animals. *Brachycladium spiciferum* as an etiologic agent. *J.Am.vet.med.Ass.* 137: 192–201.

Campbell, Charlotte C. The accuracy of serologic methods in diagnosis. *Ann.N.Y.Acad.Sci.* 89: 63–77.

Ciferri, R. *Manuale di mycologia medicale,* 2 vols. Pavia.

*Das-Gupta, S. N., Shome, S. K. & Majumdar, S. S. Medical mycology in India. *Mycopathologia* 13: 339–76.

Griffin, D. M. The re-discovery of *Gymnoascus gypseum,* the perfect state of *Microsporum gypseum.* And a note on *Trichophyton terrestre. Trans. Br.mycol.Soc.* 43: 637–42. [See also *Nature* 186: 94–5 (1960).]

Maddy, K. T., Crecelius, H. G. & Cornell, R. G. Distribution of *Coccidioides immitis* determined by testing cattle. *Publ.Health Rep.Wash.* 75: 955–62.

Negroni, P. *Micosis profundis (cutáneas y viscerales).* II. *Histoplasmosis. Histoplasmosis en la Argentina.* La Plata. [Engl.transl. *Histoplasmosis. Diagnosis and Treatment* (1965) Springfield, Ill.]

*Paldrok, H. Medical mycology in Scandinavia and Finland during a century, from 1841 to 1940. *Mycopathologia* 12: 289–348.

Segretain, G., Drouhet, E. & Mariat, F. *Diagnostique de laboratoire en mycologie médicale.* Paris.

Stevens, A. J., Saunders, C. N., Spence, J. B. & Newnham, Audrey G. Investigation into 'disease' of turkey poults. *Vet.Rec.* 72: 627–8. **Aflatoxicosis**

Sweany, H. C. *Histoplasmosis.* Springfield, Ill. [History pp. 14–39.]

Taschdjian, C. L., Burchall, J. J. & Kozinn, P. J. Rapid identification of *Candida albicans* by filamentation on serum and serum substitutes, *Am.J.dis.Child.* 99: 2; 2–5.

1961   Birmingham, D. J., Key, M. M., Tubich, G. E. & Perone, V. B. Phytotoxic bullae among celery harvesters. *Arch.Derm.Syph.Chicago* **83**: 73–87.

Blount, W. P. Turkey 'X' disease. *J.Br.Turkey Fed.* **9**: 52, 55–8.

Bridges, C. H. & Emmons, C. W. A phycomycosis of horses caused by *Hyphomyces destruens*. *J.Am.vet.med.Ass.* **138**: 579–89.

Brygoo, E. R. La mycologie médicale à Madagascar. *Arch.Inst. Pasteur Madagascar* **29**: 45–63. [See also **36**: 83–113 (1967).]

Dawson, Christine O. & Gentles, J. C. The perfect states of *Keratomyces ajelloi* Vanbreuseghem, *Trichophyton terrestre* Durie & Frey and *Microsporum nanum* Fuentes. *Sabouraudia* **1**: 49–57.

Denton, J. F., McDonough, E. S., Ajello, L. & Ausherman, R. J. Isolation of *Blastomyces dermatitidis* from soil. *Science* **133**: 1126–7.

Donomae, I. (ed.). *Studies on candidiasis*. Tokyo (Res.Comm. of Candidiasis. Japan).

Gregson, A. E. W. & La Touche, C. J. Otomycosis: a neglected disease. *J.Laryng.Otol.* **75**: 45–69.

Jelínek, V. & Sobra, K. *Veterinárini dermatologie*. Prague.

Lancaster, M. C., Jenkins, F. P. & Philip, J. M. Toxicity associated with certain samples of groundnuts. *Nature*, **192**: 1095–6.

*Randhawa, H. S., Sandhu, R. S. & Viswanathan, R. Medical mycology in India – a review of work done since 1910. *Indian J.Chest Dis.* **3**: 33–49.

Sargeant, K., O'Kelly, J., Carnaghan, R. B. A. & Allcroft, Ruth. The assay of a toxic principle in Brazilian groundnut meal. *Vet.Rec.* **73**: 1215–19.

Sargeant, K., Sheridan, Ann, O'Kelly, J. & Carnaghan, R. B. A. Toxicity associated with certain samples of groundnuts. *Nature* **192**: 1096–7.

Schoental, R. Liver changes and primary liver tumours in rats given a toxic pig diet (M.R.C. diet 18). *Br.J.Cancer* **15**: 812–15.

Stockdale, Phyllis M. *Nannizzia incurvata* gen.nov., sp.nov., a perfect state of *Microsporum gypseum* Guiart & Grigorakis. *Sabouraudia* **1**: 41–8.

1961–3 Hasenclever, H. F. & Mitchell, W. O. Antigenic studies of Candida. I. Observations on two antigenic groups of *Candida albicans*. *J.Bact.* **82**: 570–3 (1961). II, III, *ibid.* **82**: 574–7; 578–81 (1961); IV, *Sabouraudia* **2**: 201–4 (1963).

1962 Ajello, L., Georg, Lucille K., Kaplan, W. & Kaufman, L. *Laboratory manual for Medical Mycology*. edn 2. Atlanta, Ga. (PHS, CDC).

Austwick, P. K. C. The presence of *Aspergillus fumigatus* in the lungs of dairy cows. *Lab.Investigation* **11**: 1065–72.

Austwick, P. K. C. & Venn, J. A. J. Mycotic abortion in England and Wales 1954–60. *Proc.ivth.Int.Congr.Anim.Reprod. The Hague, 1961* **3**: 562–8.

Campbell, Charlotte, C., Hill, Grace B. & Falgout, B. T. *Histoplasma capsulatum* isolated from feather pillow associated with histoplasmosis in an infant. *Science* **136**: 1050–1.

English, Mary P. & Dalton, G. A. An outbreak of fungal infections of post-operative aural cavities. *J.Laryng.Otol.* **76**: 1–2. See also *ibid.* **76**: 12–21 (1962); **77**: 422–9 (1963).

*Forgacs, J. & Carll, W. T. Mycotoxicoses. *Adv.vet.Sci.* **7**: 273–382.

*Restrepo-Morendo, Angela, Calle-Velez, G., Sánchez-Arbelaéz, J. & Correa-Gonzalez, A. A review of medical mycology in Colombia, South America. *Mycopathologia* **17**: 93–110.

Smalley, E. B., Nichols, R. E., Crump, M. H. & Henning, A. A physiological disturbance in animals resulting from the ingestion of *Rhizoctonia leguminicola* infested red clover. *Phytopathology* **52**: 753.

1963   Austwick, P. K. C. & Ayerst, G. Groundnut microflora and toxicity. *Chemistry & Industry 1963*: 55–61.

Barker, S. A., Cruickshank, C. N. D. & Morris, J. A. Structure of a galactomanan-peptide allergen from *Trichophyton mentagrophytes*. *Biochim.biophys.Acta* **74**: 239–46.

English, Mary P. The saprophytic growth of keratinophilic fungi on keratin. *Sabouraudia* **2**: 115–30.

Emmons, C. W., Binford, C. H. & Utz, J. P. *Medical Mycology*. Philadelphia. [edn 3 (1977).]

Londero, A. T., Fischman, Olga & Ramos, Cecy. Animal ringworm in Brazil. *O Hospital* **63**: 259–63.

Pepys, J., Jenkins, P. A., Festenstein, G. N., Gregory, P. H., Lacey, Maureen E. & Skinner, F. A. Farmer's lung. Thermophilic actinomycetes as a source of 'farmer's lung hay' antigen. *Lancet 1963* **2**: 607–11.

Scheel, L. D., Perone, D., Larkin, R. L. & Kupel, R. E. The isolation and characterization of two phototoxic furanocoumarins (psoralens) from diseased celery. *Biochemistry* **2**: 1127–31.

Schwarz, J. & Baum, G. L. Reinfection in histoplasmosis. *Arch Path.* **75**: 475–9.

Seeliger, H. P. Immunbiologisch-serologische Nachweisverfahren bei Pilz-krankungen. In (Jadassohn's) *Handb. Haut- und Geschlechtskrankheiten* (A. Marchionini & H. Gotz, Eds) **4**: 605–734.

1964   Ajello, L. Relationship of *Histoplasma capsulatum* to avian habitats. *Publ.Health Rep.Wash.* **79**: 266–70.

Karunaratne, W. A. E. *Rhinosporidiosis in man.* London.

Moyer, D. G. & Keeler, C. Note on the culture of black piedra for cosmetic reasons. *Arch.Derm.Syph.Chicago* **89**: 436.

*Mumford, E. P. Human mycoses in the Near and Middle East. *J.trop. Med.Hyg.* **67**: 35–41.

Sarkisov, A. K. [*Mycoses and mycotoxicoses.*] Moscow. [Russ.]

Smith, C. D. & Furcolow, M. L. The demonstration of growth stimulating substances for *Histoplasma capsulatum* and *Blastomyces dermatitidis* in infusions of starling (*Sturnis vulgaris*) manure. *Mycopathologia* **22**: 73–80.

Winner, H. I. & Hurley, Rosalinde. *Candida albicans.* London. [2000 refs.]

1965   Ashley, L. M., Halver, J. E., Gardner Jr, W. K. & Wogan, G. N. Crystalline aflatoxins cause trout hepatoma. *Fed.Proc.* 24L 627.

Austwick, P. K. C. Pathogenicity in K. B. Raper & Dorothy I. Fennell, *The genus Aspergillus*, chap. 7 (pp. 82–126).

Dodge, H. J., Ajello, L. & Engelke, O. K. The association of a bird-roosting site with infection of school children by *Histoplasma capsulatum*. *Am.J.publ.Health* **55**: 1203–11.

González-Ochoa, A. Contribuciones recientes al conocimiento de la esporotrichosis. *Gac.méd.Méx.* **95**: 463–74.

*Schwarz, J. & Baum, G. L. Pioneers in the discovery of deep mycoses. *Mycopathologia* **25**: 73–81.

Sinnhuber, R. O., Wales, J. H., Engebrecht, R. H., Amend, D. F., Kray, W. D., Ayers, J. L. & Aston, W. E. Aflatoxins in cottonseed meal and hepatoma in rainbow trout. *Fed.Proc.* **24**: 627.

Van de Merwe, K. J., Steyn, P. S., Fourie, L., Scott, D. E. R. & Theron, J. J. Ochratoxin A, a toxic metabolite produced by *Aspergillus ochraceus* Wilh. *Nature* **205**: 1112–13.

Zapater, R. C. *Introducción a la micologia médica*. Buenos Aires.

1966 Converse, J. L. & Reed, R. E. Experimental epidemiology of coccidioidomycosis. *Bact.Rev.* **30**: 679–94.

Emanuel, D. A., Wenzel, F. J. & Lawton, B. R. *New Engl.J.Med.* **244**: 1413–18. Pneumonitis due to *Cryptostroma corticale* (maple-bark disease).

McFarland, R. B. Sporotrichosis revisited: 65-year follow up of the second reported case [Hektoen & Perkins, 1900, q.v.]. *Ann.intern.Med.* **65**: 363–6.

Vanbreuseghem, R. *Guide pratique de mycologie médicale et vétérinaire*. Paris. [edn 2 (with C. Vroey & M. Takashio, 1978).]

Winner, H. I. & Hurley, Rosalinde (eds). *Symposium on Candida infections*. London.

1967 Ajello, L. (ed.) *Coccidioidomycosis, the proceedings of the Second Symposium on Coccidioidomycosis, Phoenix, Ariz. 8–10 Dec. 1965*. Tucson (Univ.Ariz.Press).

*Alkiewicz, J. A. On the discovery of *Trichophyton schoenleinii* (*Achorion schoenleinii*). *Mycopathologia* **33**: 28–32.

Connole, M. D. & Johnston, L. A. Y. A review of animal mycoses in Australia. *Vet.Bull.* **37**: 145–53.

Drouhet, E., Marcel, M. & Labonde, J. Flore dermatophytique des picines. *Bull Soc.franç.Dermat.Syph.* **74**: 719–24.

Heim, R., Cailleux, R., Wasson, R. G. & Thévenard, P. *Nouvelle investigations sur les champignons hallucinogènes*. Paris (Mus.Nat.Hist.Natur.)

Hugh-Jones, M. E. & Austwick, P. K. C. Epidemiological studies on bovine mycotic abortion. I. The effect of the climate on incidence. *Vet.Rec.* **81**: 273–6.

Hurley, Rosalinde. The pathogenic Candida species: a review. *Rev.med. vet.Mycol.* **6**: 159–76.

Lacaz, C. da Silva. *Compêndio de micologia medica*. São Paulo. [edn 7 (with E. Porto & J. E. Martins), *Micologia medica* (1984).]

Rifkin, D., Marchioro, T. L., Schenck, S. A. & Hill, R. B. Systemic fungal infections complicating renal transplantation and immunosuppressive therapy. *Am.J.Med.* **43**: 28–38.

*Shanks, S. C. Vale epilatio. X-ray epilation of the scalp at Goldie Leigh Hospital. Woolwich (1922–58). *Br.J.Derm.* **79**: 237–8.

Strand, R. D., Neuhauser, E. B. D. & Sornberger, C. F. Lycoperdonosis. *New Engl.J.Med.* **227**: 89–91.

Tosh, F. E., Weeks, R. J., Pfeiffer, F. R., Hendricks, S. L., Greer, D. L. & Chin, T. D. Y. The use of formalin to kill *Histoplasma capsulatum* at an epidemic site *Am.J.Epidem.* **85**: 259–65.

Winn, W. A. A working classification of coccidioidomycosis and its application to therapy. In Ajello (1967): 3–10.

1968   Cross, T., Maciver, Ann M. & Lacey, J. The thermophilic actinomycetes of mouldy hay: *Micropolyspora faeni* sp.nov. *J.gen.Microbial.* **50**: 351–9.

Durie, E. Beatrix & Frey, Dorothea. Fungus infections of the skin in Australia. *Austral.J.Derm.* **9**: 232–6.

English, Mary P. The developmental morphology of the perforating organs and eroding mycelium of dermatophytes. *Sabouraudia* **6**: 218–27.

Kubička, J. Traitement des empoisonnements fongiques phalloidiens en Tchecoslovacuie. *Acta mycol.Warsaw* **4**: 373–7.

Lacey, J. The microflora of fodders associated with bovine respiratory disease. *J.gen.Microbiol.* **51**: 173–7.

Moreau, C. *Moisissures toxiques dans l'alimentation.* Paris. [edn 2 (1974).]

Smith, J. M. B. Animal mycoses in New Zealand. *Mycopathologia* **34**: 323–6.

Vic-Dupont, V., Coulaud, J. P. & Delrieu, F. Les septicémies à 'Candida'. Aspects étiologiques, cliniques et thérapeutiques. D'après 30 observations. *Presse méd.* **76**: 747–50.

*Wasson, R. G. *Soma, the divine mushroom of immortality.* Folio. The Hague. [Reprint, 8vo (1971).]

Wieland, T. Poisoning principles of mushrooms of the genus *Amanita*. *Science* **159**: 946–52.

1969   Bronner, Marcell & Bronner, Max. *Actinomycosis.* Bristol.

Goldblatt, L. A. (ed.). *Aflatoxin. Scientific background, control, and implications.* New York & London.

Jellison, W. L. *Adiaspiromycosis* (= *Haplomycosis*). Missoula, Montana.

*Lepper, A. W. D. Immunological aspects of dermatomycoses in animals and man. *Rev.med.vet.Mycol.* **6**: 435–46.

Lurie, H. I. & Still, W. I. S. The 'capsule' of *Sporotrichum schenckii* and the evolution of the asteroid body. *Sabouradia* **7**: 64–70.

1970   *Bové, F. J. *The story of ergot.* Basel.

*Frey, Dorothea & Durie, E. Beatrix. Deep mycoses reported from Australia and New Guinea during the years 1956 to 1969. *Med.J.Austral.* **57**: 1117–23.

Krogh, P., Hasselager, E. & Friis, P. Studies on fungal nepthrotoxicity. 2. Isolation of two nephrotoxic compounds from *Penicillium viridicatum* Westling. Citrinin and oxalic acid. *Acta Path.Microbiol.Scand.* B **78**: 401–13.

Lehner, T. & Ward, R. G. Iatrogenic oral candidosis. *Br.J.Derm.* **83**: 161–6.

Roberts, J. A., Counts, J. M. & Crecelius, H. G. Production *in vitro* of *Coccidioides immitis* spherules and endospores as a diagnostic aid. *Am.Rev.resp.Dis.* **102**: 811–13.

Balows, A. (ed.). *Histoplasmosis. Proceedings of the Second National Conference* [Oct. 1969.] Springfield. Ill.

1971   Buechner, H. A. (ed.) *Management of fungus diseases of the lungs.* Springfield, Ill.

Lacey, J. *Thermoactinomyces sacchari* sp.nov., a thermophilic actinomycete causing bagassosis. *J.gen.Microbiol.* **66**: 327–38.

Migaki, G., Valerio, M. G., Irvine, B. & Garner, F. M. Lobo's disease in an Atlantic bottle-nosed dolphin [*Tursiops truncatus*]. *J.Am.vet.med.Ass.* **159**: 578–82.

O'Meara, B. & Wheelwright, C. *A Bibliography of Avian Mycoses (partially annotated)*, edn 3. Orono (Univ. Maine). [1016 refs.]

Pirie, H. M., Dawson, Christine O., Breeze, R. G., Wiseman, A. & Hamilton, J. A bovine disease similar to farmer's lung: extrinsic allergic alveolitis. *Vet.Rec.* **88**: 346–51.

1971–   Ciegler, A., Kadis, S. & Ajl, S. (eds). *Microbial toxins. A compre-*
72   *hensive treatise.* 6, *Fungal toxins,* 1971. Kadis, Ciegler & Ajl (eds) 7, *Algal and fungal toxins,* 1971; 8, *Fungal toxins,* 1972. New York.

1972   *Ajello, L. (a) The mycoses of Oceania. *Mycopathologia* **46**: 87–95. (b)* Paracoccidiodomycosis: a historical review. In *Proceedings of the First Pan American Symposium* PAHO WHO: 3–10.

Al-Doory, Y. *Chromomycosis.* Missoula, Montana.

François, J. & Rysselaere, M. *Oculomycosis.* Springfield, Ill.

*Higgs, Janet M. Muco-cutaneous candidiasis: Historical aspects. *Trans. St John's Hosp.Derm.Soc.* **59**: 175–94.

Hyde, H. A. Atmospheric pollen and spores in relation to allergy. I. *Clin.Allergy* **2**: 153–79 [*c.* 200 refs].

Jungerman, P. F. & Schwartzman, R. M. *Veterinary medical mycology.* Philadelphia.

Lowy, B. Mushroom symbolism in Maya codices. *Mycologia* **64**: 816–21. [See also *Revista Interamerica Review* **5**: 110–18, 1975.]

Pirie, H. M., Dawson, Christine O., Breeze, R. G., Selman, I. E. & Wiseman, A. Precipitans to *Micropolyspora faeni* in the adult cattle of selected herds in Scotland and north-west England. *Clin.Allergy* **2**: 181–7.

*Sran, H. S., Narula, I. M. S., Agarwal, R. K. & Joshi, K. R. History of mycetoma. *Indian J.Hist.Med.* **17**: 1–7.

1973   De Vries, G. A. & Laarman, J. J. A case of Lobo's disease in the dolphin (*Sotalia guianensis*). *Aquatic Mammals* **1**: 26–33.

Gregory, P. H. *Microbiology of the atmosphere*, edn 2. London [edn 1, 1961.] [Historical introduction pp. 1–14.]

Lacey, J. The air spora of a Portuguese cork factory. *Ann.occup.Hyg.* **16**: 223–30.

Mahgoub, El Sheikh & Murray, I. G. *Mycetoma.* London.

Powell, K. E., Hammerman, K. J., Dahl, B. A. & Tosh, F. E. Acute reinfection pulmonary histoplasmosis. A report of six cases. *Ann.Rev.resp.Dis.* **107**: 374–8.

Schlueter, D. P. 'Cheesewasher's disease': a new occupational hazard. *Ann.internal Med.* **78**: 606.

1974 Ajello, L. Natural history of the dermatophytes and related fungi. *Mycopathologia* **53**: 93–110.

Austwick, P. K. C. & Copland, J. W. Swamp cancer. *Nature* **250**: 84.

Purchase, I. F. H. (ed.). *Mycotoxins.* Amsterdam.

*Scholer, H. J. Stellung und Bedeutung der Mykosen unter den menischlichen Infektionskrankheiten. *Pathologia et Microbiologia* **41**: 199–231.

Sheklakov, N. D. & Milich, M. V. *Mycoses in man.* Moscow. [Transl. from Russian (1970 edn) by D. A. Myshne.]

1975

Austwick, P. K. C. Environmental aspects of *Mortierella wolfii* infection in cattle. *N.Z.J.agric.Res.* **19**: 25–33.

*Bloch, M., Quintanilla, Lucrecia & Rivera, H. Systemic mycosis in El Salvador. *Rev.Inst.Investigaciones Medicas* **4**: 23–57.

Caldwell, D. K., Caldwell, Melba C., Woodward, J. C., Ajello, L., Kaplan, W. & McClure, H. M. Lobomycosis as a disease of the Atlantic bottlenosed dolphin (*Tursiops truncatus* Montagu, 1821). *Am.J.trop.Med.Hyg.* **24**: 105–14.

Chick, E. W., Balows, A. & Furcolow, M. L. (eds). *Opportunist fungal infections.* Springfield, Ill.

Hatfield, G. M. & Schaumberg, J. P. Isolation and structural studies on coprine, the disulfiram-like constituent of *Coprinus atramentarius*. *Lloydia* **38**: 489–96. Coprine

Hempel H. & Goodman, N. L. Rapid conversion of *Histoplasma capsulatum*, *Blastomyces dermatididis* and *Sporothrix schenckii* in tissue culture. *J.clin.Microbiol.* **1**: 420–4.

Smith, L. P. & Austwick, P. K. C. Effect of weather on the quality of wool in Great Britain. *Vet.Rec.* **96**: 246–8.

1976 *Ainsworth, G. C. *Introduction to the history of mycology.* Cambridge.

Evans, E. G. V. (ed). *Serology of fungal infections and farmer's lung disease. A laboratory manual.* Leeds (Br.Soc.Mycopath.)

Sarkisov, A. K. Prophylaxie spécifique de la trichophytose des jeunes bovins. *Bull.Office internat.Épizooties* (FAO) **85**: 481–8.

1977 Ajello, L. (a)*Milestones in the history of medical mycology: the dermatophytes. In Iwata (1977a): 3–11. (b)(ed.) *Coccidioidomycosis. Current clinical and diagnostic status.* New York. [= Rep. 3rd Internat. Coccidioidomycosis Symp. (1976).]

Al-Doory, Y. (ed). *The epidemiology of human mycotic diseases.* Springfield, Ill.

Blyth, W., Grant, J. W. B., Blackadder, E. S. & Greenberg, M. Fungal antigens as a source of sensitization and respiratory disease in Scottish maltworkers. *Clin.Allergy* 7: 549–62.

Edwards, J. H. Humidifier fever. *Thorax* 32: 653–63.

Iwata, K. (a) (ed.). *Recent advances in medical and veterinary mycology.* Baltimore. [Proc.6th. Internat.Congr. of ISHAM, Tokyo (1975).] (b) *The history of the Japanese Society for Medical Mycology: from the year of its foundation to the 20th Anniversary. *Jap.J.med.Mycol.* 18: 244–62.

Lincoff, G. & Mitchell, D. H. *Toxic and hallucinogenic mushroom poisoning. A handbook for physicians and mushroom hunters.* New York.

Palmer, D. F. & Kaufman, L., Kaplan, W. & Cavallaro, J. J. *Serodiagnosis of mycotic disease.* Springfield, Ill.

1977–8 Wyllie, T. D. & Morehouse, L. G. (eds). *Mycotoxic fungi, mycotoxins, mycotoxicoses. An encyclopedic handbook.* 1 (*Mycotoxic fungi and chemistry of mycotoxins*), 1977: 2 (*Mycotoxicoses of domestic and laboratory animals, poultry, and aquatic invertebrates and vertebrates*); 3 (*Mycotoxicoses of man and plants; mycotoxin control and regulatory aspects*), 1978. New York & Basel.

1978 *Ainsworth, G. C. The Medical Research Council's Medical Mycology Committee (1943–69). A chapter in the history of medical mycology in the United Kingdom. *Sabouraudia* 16: 1–7.

Heathcote, J. G. & Hibbert, J. R. *Aflatoxins: chemical and biological aspects.* Amsterdam.

Kashkin, P. N. & Sheklakov, N. D. [*Guide to medical mycology.*] Moscow. [Russ.]

Rumack, B. H. & Salzman, E. (eds). *Mushroom poisoning: diagnosis and treatment.* West Palm Beach, Fla.

Willoughby, L. G. Saprolegniasis of salmonid fish in Windermere: a critical analysis. *J.Fish Dis.* 1: 51–67.

1979 Bennett, J. E. *et al.* [15 authors]. A comparison of amphotericin B alone and combined with flucytosine in the treatment of cryptococcal meningitis. *New Engl.J.Med.* 301: 126–31.

Frey, Dorothea, Oldfield, R. J. & Bridger, R. C. *A colour atlas of pathogenic fungi.* London.

*Hesseltine, C. W. Introduction, definition, and history of mycotoxins of importance to animal production. In *Interactions of mycotoxins in animal production*: 3–15. Washington, DC (Nat.Acad.Sci.).

Lutwick, L. I., Rytel, M. W., Peña Yanez, J., Galgiani, J. N. & Stevens, D. A. Deep infections due to *Petriellidium boydii* treated with miconazole. *J.Am.med.Ass.* 241: 272–3.

Odds, F. *Candida and Candidosis.* Leicester Univ. Press. [2265 refs.]

Salfelder, K., Schwarz, J. & Sauerteig, E. *Colour atlas of deep mycoses in man.* Stuttgart.

1980 Chandler, F. W., Kaplan, W. & Ajello, L. *A color atlas and textbook of the histopathology of mycotic disease.* London.

Domer, Judith, E. & Moser, S. A. Histoplasmosis – a review. *Rev.med.vet.Mycol.* 15: 159–82.

McGinnis, M. R. *Laboratory handbook of medical mycology.* New York.

*Recalde, F. Micosis: bibliografíca. Autores nacionales. *Revista Paraguaya de Microbiológica* **15**: 41–3.

Speller, D. C. E. (ed.). *Antifungal chemotherapy.* Chichester, UK.

Stevens, D. A. (ed.). *Coccidioidomycosis. A text.* New York. [History pp. 1–20.]

1981   *Baldwin, R. S. *The fungus fighters.* Cornell Univ. Press. [Rachael Brown, Elizabeth Hazen.]

Dumont, Anne-Marie, Chennebault, Jean-Marie, Alquier, P. & Jardel, H. Management of *Amanita phalloides* poisoning by Bastien's regimen. *Lancet 1981* **1**: 722.

Fletcher, L. R. & Harvey, I. C. An association of a *Lolium* endophyte with ryegrass staggers. *N.Z.vet.J.* **29**: 185–6.

Gallagher, R. T., White, E. P. & Mortimer, P. H. Ryegrass staggers: isolation of potent neurotoxins lolitrem A and lolitrem B from staggers-producing pastures. *N.Z.vet.J.* **29**: 189–90.

*Hornstein, O. P. Laudatio auf Professor Dr. Dr.h.c. Hans Michael Götz. *Mykosen* **24**: 650–2.

*Schadewalt, H. Anfänge der Medizinischen Mykologie in Deutschland. *Mykosen* **24**: 654–7.

1982   Del Negro, G., Lacaz, C. da Silva & Fiorillo, A. M. (eds). *Paracoccidioidomicose. Blastomicose Sul-americana.* São Paulo.

*Eliasson, O. Farmer's lung disease: a new historical perspective from Iceland. *J.Hist.Med.* **37**: 440–3.

*Grmek, M. D. Intoxication par les champignons dans l'antiquité Grecque et Latine. In *Littér. Méd.Soc., Simples et drogues,* Univ. Nantes, No. 4: 17–52.

International nomenclature of diseases. 2. Infectious diseases. Part 2. *Mycoses.* Geneva (CIOMS).

Klastersky, J. (ed.). *Infections in cancer patients.* New York.

McGinnis, M. R., D'Amato, R. F. & Land, G. *Pictorial handbook of medically important fungi and aerobic actinomycetes.* New York.

McGinnis, M. R., Padhye, A. A. & Ajello, L. *Pseudallescheria* Negroni & Fischer, 1943 and its later synonym *Petriellidium* Malloch, 1970. *Mycotaxon* **14**: 94–102.

Plotzker, R., Jensen, D. M. & Payne, J. A. *Amanita virosa* acute hepatic necrosis: treatment with thioctic acid. *Am.J.med.Sci.* **283**: 79–82.

Rippon, J. W. *Medical mycology. The pathogenic fungi and the pathogenic actinomycetes,* edn 2. Philadelphia. [edn 1, 1974.]

Warnock, D. W. & Richardson, M. D. (eds). *Fungal infection in the compromised patient.* Chichester, UK.

1983   *Ainsworth, G. C. & Stockdale, Phyllis M. Landmarks in medical and veterinary mycology. *Rev.med.vet.Mycol.* **18**: 9–18.

DiSalvo, A. F. (ed.). *Occupational mycoses.* Philadelphia.

*Lacaz, C. da Silva. História da micologia médica no Brasil. *Ann.bras.Derm.* **58**: 265–70.

Ueno, Y. (ed.). *Trichothecenes. Chemical, biological and toxicological aspects.* Amsterdam

1983–5 Howard, D. H. (ed.). *Fungi pathogenic for humans and animals,* 3 vols. New York & Basel.

1984 *Ainsworth, G. C. & Stockdale, Phyllis M. Biographical notices of deceased medical and veterinary mycologists. *Rev.med.vet.Mycol.* **19**: 1–13.

Al-Doory, Y. & Domson, Joanne F. (eds). *Mould allergy.* Philadelphia.

Margot, P., Farquhar, G. & Watling, R. Identification of toxic mushrooms and toadstools (agarics) – an on-line identification programme. In R. Alkin & F. A. Bisby (eds.), *Databases in systematics,* London.

*Pereiro Miguens, M. (a) Revisíon de la micología Española desde 1909 á 1983. (Especialmente médica y veterinária). *Revista Iberica Micol.* **1**: 45–59. (b) *Pasado, presente y futuro de la micologia en España.* Trabo presentado en la 2a Reunión Conjunta de Micología celebrado en Bellaterra (Barcelona) los dias 31 de Mayo, 1 y 2 Junio de 1984. [Mimeographed.]

Roberts, S. O. B., Hay, R. J. & Mackenzie, D. W. R. *A clinician's guide to fungal disease.* New York & Basel.

1985 Bodey, G. P. & Fainstein, V. (eds). *Candidiasis.* New York.

*Huntington, R. W. Four great coccidioidomycologists: William Ophuls (1871–1933), Myrnie Gifford (1892–1966), Charles Edward Smith (1904–1967) and William A. Winn (1903–1967). *Sabouraudia* **23**: 361–70.

*Seeliger, H. P. R. The discovery of *Achorion schoenleinii.* Facts and 'stories'. *Mykosen* **28**: 161–82.

NAMES INDEX

SUBJECT INDEX

224